P9-DJA-055

Balancing Pregnancy with Pre-Existing Diabetes

DATE DUE

SEP 2 6 2011			

Demco, Inc. 38-293

Balancing Pregnancy with Pre-Existing Diabetes

Healthy Mom, Healthy Baby

Cheryl Alkon

618.3
A415

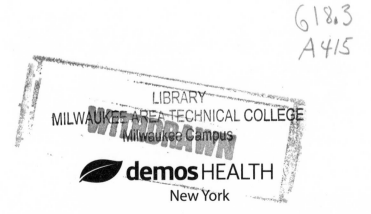

LIBRARY
MILWAUKEE AREA TECHNICAL COLLEGE
Milwaukee Campus
WITHDRAWN

demosHEALTH

New York

Acquisitions Editor: Noreen Henson
Cover Design: Carlos Maldonado
Compositor: Newgen North America
Printer: Hamilton Printing

Visit our website at www.demosmedpub.com

© 2010 Demos Medical Publishing, LLC. All rights reserved. This book is protected by copyright. No part of it may be reproduced, stored in a retrieval system, or transmitted in any form or by any means, electronic, mechanical, photocopying, recording, or otherwise, without the prior written permission of the publisher.

Medical information provided by Demos Health, in the absence of a visit with a healthcare professional, must be considered as an educational service only. This book is not designed to replace a physician's independent judgment about the appropriateness or risks of a procedure or therapy for a given patient. Our purpose is to provide you with information that will help you make your own healthcare decisions.

The information and opinions provided here are believed to be accurate and sound, based on the best judgment available to the authors, editors, and publisher, but readers who fail to consult appropriate health authorities assume the risk of any injuries. The publisher is not responsible for errors or omissions. The editors and publisher welcome any reader to report to the publisher any discrepancies or inaccuracies noticed.

Library of Congress Cataloging-in-Publication Data

Alkon, Cheryl.
  Balancing pregnancy with pre-existing diabetes : healthy mom, healthy baby / Cheryl Alkon.
      p. cm.
  Includes bibliographical references and index.
  ISBN 978-1-932603-32-3
  1. Diabetes in pregnancy—Popular works. I. Title.
  RG580.D5A45 2010
  618.3—dc22   2009053469

Special discounts on bulk quantities of Demos Health books are available to corporations, professional associations, pharmaceutical companies, health care organizations, and other qualifying groups. For details, please contact:

Special Sales Department
Demos Medical Publishing
11 W. 42nd Street
New York, NY 10036
Phone: 800–532–8663 or 212–683–0072
Fax: 212–941–7842
E-mail: rsantana@demosmedpub.com

Made in the United States of America

10 11 12   13   5 4 3 2 1

To Dave and Ethan, my wonderful family,
who make everything worthwhile.

To Shanie and Bert, my beloved Mom and Dad,
who made everything possible.

Contents

Foreword

"Why do I need to control my blood sugars before I become pregnant?" "What will this high blood sugar do to my baby now that I am pregnant?" "Why do I need to see my eye doctor during pregnancy?" "What can I eat now that I am pregnant?" Cheryl Alkon and her network of women with diabetes offer their stories and advice to help answer these and more questions from a wide variety of perspectives.

This thoughtful and comprehensive book takes you step by step from planning your pregnancy, to that moment when you see the two lines on your home pregnancy test, to meal planning when you have morning sickness, to understanding the recommended obstetric testing, to the fine points of controlling your blood glucose levels during the long haul of pregnancy, labor, and delivery and while you are breast-feeding. Infertility and miscarriage can occur even if you do everything you possibly can, and this book helps you understand why.

The experiences and viewpoints of many women are shared throughout this book. Together, they offer valuable personal and collective knowledge about how to optimize diabetes control and improve outcomes for all women and their babies. They have been there; you may be in the same place as they were at each step but may not yet have found someone with whom to share your perspectives or questions. You may not agree with all of the choices that these women made regarding their diabetes self-management before, during, and after pregnancy, but many approaches and insights are offered, and readers can reflect on these and discuss them with their own health care providers.

   Most important is that even if you are highly motivated to control your diabetes for your baby, your diabetes control will never be perfect. You will feel guilt, fear, or sadness about something during your pregnancy. You are not alone, and this book is a great way to connect with other women who have done this before with success. Even if things go well for you in achieving pregnancy and caring for yourself and your baby during pregnancy and after, you may love to hear other patients' stories about their experiences.

   This book is the first practical peer reference for women with preconception diabetes to be published.

Florence Brown, MD
Tamara Takoudes, MD
Codirectors
Joslin-Beth Israel Deaconess Medical Center
Diabetes and Pregnancy Program
Boston, Massachusetts

You Can Definitely
Do This—And Do It Well

So you want to have a kid, but you already have a nagging, never-ending, highly demanding thing in your life: your diabetes. Like a child, diabetes requires constant maintenance and vigilance to make sure everything's running as smoothly as possible. Unlike a child, though, diabetes never really takes a nap or hangs out with the babysitter to give you a moment's peace.

But don't let that stop you.

Search medical journals or go online and Google "diabetes and pregnancy," and what you'll find will likely freak you out. Uncontrolled blood sugars can lead to complications. Early inductions. Premature lungs. Big babies. Small babies. Birth defects.

Your research might make you think it's a miracle that anyone with diabetes ever had a healthy pregnancy. Is every pregnancy with diabetes problematic? Are the kids of all these moms with diabetes doomed to a lifetime of horrible problems due to bathing in a sweet soup while in utero?

The answer to these questions is no. In talking to dozens of women about all aspects of pregnancy with type 1 and type 2 diabetes, and ultimately managing my own healthy type 1 pregnancy, I've learned (and lived) the insider story from those who delivered healthy babies before me. Some women experienced complications, but they've shared how they handled those challenges and how any woman with diabetes can adapt to deal with them if they occur.

"There are a lot of women with type 1 diabetes who have been told at some point in their lives that they couldn't have children," said Ian

Grable, MD, MPH, director of the Center for Maternal and Fetal Health at NorthShore University HealthSystem in the Chicago (Illinois) area. "Many women who have been diabetic a long time were told this by general medicine doctors or family practitioners. In this day and age, while being followed by a maternal/fetal medicine specialist, an obstetrician, and an endocrinologist with an expertise in pregnancy, pregnancy can be safe. A healthy pregnancy, with delivery at or near term, is possible."

I'm here to share with you what I have learned along the way and to help you manage the sweetness within yourself.

Acknowledgments

Reading is a solitary pursuit, but creating a book sure isn't. While the writing itself took place in my silent house, the information offered through countless e-mails, phone calls, and faxes from many other people provided a chatty chorus of insight and made this work stronger and more comprehensive.

Blogging has been an integral component of this book, and online communities have supplied most of the voices that fill it. Thank you to everyone who has read, commented on, or linked to my blog, "Managing the Sweetness Within." Writing and maintaining my blog about my efforts to get and stay pregnant with type 1 diabetes helped me develop a voice for this book, and blog feedback helped convince people that this kind of guide was sorely needed and would be welcomed. Thank you to the more than 100 women who found me, through my blog and other online diabetes resources, and wanted to answer questions about their experiences with diabetes, conception, pregnancy, infertility, pregnancy loss, and parenthood. Space doesn't allow me to write out all your names, but I am thanking each of you individually in my head.

Many thanks go to Kim Kavin, Laurie Edwards, and Janice Hopkins Tanne, who read early versions of my book proposal and gave priceless advice about how to make it stronger and more marketable. Again, major props to Kim, who proofread every word of the final draft with a fantastic eye for detail. Thank you to Melissa Ford, who sent me her terrific list of potential agents when I was ready to find one of my own. The agent I signed with, Molly Lyons of Joelle Delbourgo Associates, saw this project for what it was and was an ardent champion without wanting to change its scope or focus significantly. Noreen Henson at Demos Medical Publishing was an enthusiastic editor who also understood what this project was about and continually advocated for it. Molly Morrison and her team at Newgen North America helped polish my prose to make everything crystal clear.

Many doctors and other health professionals lent their expertise to give this book a solid foundation in medicine. My thanks and gratitude go to Ian Grable, Emmy Suhl, Deborah Schlossman, Lonnie Morris, Judith Maloni, Gary Scheiner, John Walsh, Sheri Colberg, Jacqueline Shahar, Michael See, Carol Levy, Stefanie Antunes, Michael J. Haller, Lois Jovanovič, Margaret Franciscus, H.-Michael Dosch, Katy Backes Kozhimannil, and Nanette Santoro.

I couldn't have had my son without Mary Beth Bahren, Flo Brown, and Tamara Takoudes; likewise, I couldn't have written this book without them. A huge thank you goes to this fabulous trio of women, who reviewed the book chapter by chapter, answered countless questions, and championed this project every step of the way.

My excellent family and friends have supported this project for many years, from conception to publication. They have cheered me on, from when I first thought about doing a book like this, to writing the proposal, to finding an agent, to commenting on every Facebook update I posted about completed chapters and author photo choices. Thanks too to those who offered to buy my book—even though some of them were neither pregnant nor living with diabetes. Much love and gratitude go to my family, Charlotte and Bert Alkon; Joe, Rebecca, and Jake Alkon; Cynthia Duncan; Susan and Justin Duncan; and Ruth, Brian, Andrew, and Joshua Weiner, and to my posse of diabetic pals, particularly those who contributed to this book, including Abby Nagel, Sasha Boak-Kelly, and Rachel Richer.

For additional fantastic friend support, thanks to Katie Kendall, Alicia Salmoni, Wendy Ross, Michelle Badash, Kara Rice, Karla Armenoff, Tina Giambro, Michelle Wilen, and also to the rest of the Girl Scout crew, the Mah Jong mavens, my New Mom friends, Chaverimers, the New York/Brandeis/Columbia crowd, and my Tri buddies. You all rock.

And finally, none of this would have been possible, or even worth writing about, were it not for my handy and handsome husband, David

Duncan, and our fantastic son, Ethan. They have provided the material for this book, the motivation to continue, and love and support through the late nights, the early mornings, the long months, and the (sometimes) short tempers. It is because of them that this book exists.

The Early Days

1

Recommendations for Trying to Conceive: If You Can, You've Gotta Plan

As a woman with long-term type 1 diabetes, I know this disease intimately. Reading this with type 1? Hi—you are my people. Type 1 is very-much-insulin-dependent, ain't-going-away-with-weight-loss-or-after-the-kid-is-born diabetes. Type 1, despite what much of the mass media or well-meaning but clueless people will tell you, is a separate condition from the far more common type 2 diabetes or gestational diabetes. Type 2 and gestational diabetes get a lot more attention when the generic term "diabetes" is thrown around, but type 1s have many specific experiences and elements that just don't apply to those other folks. At the same time, to stay within the tight recommended blood sugar ranges before conception and during pregnancy, most if not all type 2 women are told to start taking insulin regularly, to watch (or continue to watch) their food intake strictly, and to juggle exercise with taking insulin. During pregnancy, type 1s and type 2s are dealing with many of the same issues of up-and-down blood sugars, the need to match insulin doses to carbohydrate intake, low blood sugars that require immediate treatment, and so on. Gestationals, on the other hand, don't even learn about diabetes until they're halfway through their pregnancies. This book focuses solely on those of us with pre-existing, rather than gestational, diabetes. We're in it for the long haul.

A quick refresher: type 1 diabetes is an autoimmune disease that occurs when the body doesn't produce insulin; type 2 diabetes occurs when the body becomes insulin resistant. Insulin is a hormone that helps your body get the most out of food, making sure nutrients get to where they need to go. When a nondiabetic eats, say, a slice of bread, the pancreas, an organ in the abdomen, automatically secretes precisely the right amount of insulin to convert the bread's vitamins and minerals into nutrition.

The body with diabetes isn't so efficient. Some people don't make any insulin at all (hello, type 1); others have to make do with a compromised amount of insulin, either all the time (welcome, type 2) or only during pregnancy (howdy, gestational). There are also a number of people who don't fall into these categories, who call themselves a mix between type 1 and type 2 (latent autoimmune diabetes in adults—a mouthful, but hi).

If you're type 1, you get insulin into your body through injections or an insulin pump. If you're type 2, you may have treated your diabetes by taking pills that help your body maximize the amount of insulin it produces to manage your blood sugars. Or you may have injected or infused insulin through a pump. Either way, women with diabetes experience a unique adventure when it comes to planning, managing, and ultimately completing a successful pregnancy. It's a marathon, not a sprint. A pregnant woman with diabetes must pay extensive attention to an odd blend of details about insulin, blood sugars, diet, exercise, fetal development, prenatal tests, countless doctor's appointments, and more, until her child finally arrives.

Whew! Tired yet?

Finding the Right Doctors

Let's say you're reading this book and you're not pregnant (if you are, skip ahead to Chapter 2). You live with diabetes. If you're type 1, you inject insulin or rock the insulin pump. If you're type 2, you might do those things or maybe you pop some oral meds or simply try to keep it all together by eating right and exercising (and you know that's not so simple). Either you're a carb counter or you try to follow an exchange diet of carbs, proteins, and fats. Your fingers are punctured with pinpricks to determine your blood sugar levels. You want to get pregnant and have a healthy baby.

Your first decision should be to find and meet with an endocrinologist a few months before you want to become pregnant, to talk specifically about pre-pregnancy diabetes management. As a woman with diabetes, you're probably already seeing an endo regularly. Ideally, this person is up to date on the latest research about diabetes and pregnancy; knows all about insulin pumps, continuous glucose monitors (CGMs), the latest insulins, and other drugs; and is familiar with emerging technologies and new medications for diabetes management.

If you're not seeing an endo (because you don't like doctors or you don't make time or you live somewhere where endos aren't plentiful) or you're being seen by an internist who isn't intimate with pregnancy with your diabetes type, you should do whatever you can to find a good diabetes doc or an internist or a certified physician's assistant who *really* knows diabetes inside and out. This person will work with you so that you can have a healthy life before pregnancy and a healthy pregnancy. Trust me on this: pregnancy is not the time to go it alone. You will likely have to see this person many times while you're trying to conceive. A good endocrinologist—or the best equivalent you can find in your area—can help you fine-tune your diabetes management every step of the way.

It's great if your endo works closely with a high-risk obstetrician/gynecologist (OB/GYN), a maternal/fetal medicine specialist, or a perinatologist who is also up to date on pregnancy with diabetes and knows the importance of tight blood sugar management. Yes, as women with diabetes, we're considered high risk. Don't let that scare you, though. Plenty of us have healthy kids and stay healthy ourselves. And it's not just the diabetes that makes some of us high risk. Women aged 35 and older, and those carrying multiples at any age, are also considered high risk. There's plenty of company in the high-risk category, and, again, many of us go on to have healthy babies.

If you're working with a regular obstetrician, who may not be closely familiar with pre-existing diabetes, educate yourself as much as possible about the condition and its effects on pregnancy. Some docs may think "all women with diabetes are the same" and have outdated notions about what people with diabetes can eat, or they might say something like "Diabetic moms always have cesarean deliveries." (Hello—totally not true.) Having your endocrinologist as an ally can help you to determine what's crucial for the health of your kid-to-be and yourself as the future mom with diabetes and to recognize old-school thinking. With tight blood sugar control, your chances of complications are the same as those of any pregnant woman without diabetes.

Questions to Ask When Meeting With a Potential Doctor Pre-Pregnancy

- Have you done this before? How many other pregnant women with type 1 or type 2 have you seen through their entire pregnancy?

- What's your style? How often do you see pregnant type 1 or type 2 patients? What if I have questions between my appointments—do you answer them by e-mail or phone? Do you expect me to fax or e-mail you logs of blood sugars, insulin, and food intake? How often? How soon can I expect a response from you?

- How will you work with me during this pregnancy? (As a patient, consider what kind of doctor personality helps you best. Maintaining tight control can be tough. If you and your doctor don't mesh well, it could be a long nine months.)

- What other health care professionals, such as a nutritionist, a high-risk OB/GYN, a certified diabetes educator (CDE), an eye doctor who specializes in retinopathy, or a nephrologist for kidney issues, do you typically work with for your patients with diabetes?

Plan Before Conceiving

Tight blood sugar control is what it's all about. It is the foundation of a healthy pregnancy with diabetes. In brief, the closer your blood sugars are to a nondiabetic's, the lower your chances are of having a baby with health problems. These problems include birth defects and macrosomia—your baby being too big and fat, which can cause problems during delivery and may later lead to a type 2 diabetes diagnosis.

The key thing about tight control is that you have to be in command of your blood sugars during the earliest days and weeks of your pregnancy. This is the crucial period when your baby is developing major body parts and when many women don't even know that they're pregnant. It's much healthier for you and your baby if you maintain tight control over your numbers as if you were pregnant, until you can test a few weeks later and know for sure. The baby's brain, spinal cord, heart, and other organs are all forming early on, and tight numbers early on will help ensure that those body parts develop as they should. Later, that same tight control might help lower your chances of a miscarriage or stillbirth. But for now, keeping the sugars in line means your baby's body will form as it is supposed to, even if you don't know for sure that you conceived this month.

Okay, so control is important. What are we talking about?

- Maintain tight blood sugars (60–150 mg/dL) before and during pregnancy.

- Make sure your hemoglobin A1c number (the average of your blood sugar readings for the past two to three months) is below a certain target (typically, 5.0–6.9 percent).

Here's how it all breaks down:

Recommended Blood Sugars (mg/dL)[1]

	Before meal	1 hour after meal	Before bed
When trying to conceive	70–110	<150	100–140
During pregnancy	60–99	<120–140	100–140

Source: see Notes (page 241).

Of course, your doctor might have other thoughts, but these are the general numbers to target.

The following table explains what your A1c numbers mean:

What Your A1c Numbers Mean[2]

A1c (%)	Estimated average glucose numbers (mg/dL)
4.0	68
4.5	82
5.0	97
5.5	111
6.0	126
6.5	140
7.0	154
7.5	169
8.0	183
8.5	197
9.0	212

© 2009 American Diabetes Association, from http://professional.diabetes.org. Reprinted with permission from The American Diabetes Association.

Bringing Your A1c Levels Down

Once you've talked to your docs about wanting to get pregnant, you'll have to walk the walk. No, I don't mean having unprotected sex yet, though you'll get there. I mean bringing your A1cs within the recommended range. The American Diabetes Association and many docs will tell you to get your A1c under 7 percent, which corresponds to an average blood sugar level of around 154 mg/dL or lower. Danish research published in the professional journal *Diabetes Care* in June 2009 found that the risks of a bad pregnancy outcome, such as a baby being born with a serious birth defect or an infant dying soon after birth, were no higher than for the general nondiabetic population if women with diabetes had A1cs of 6.9 percent or lower.[3] (Women with A1cs of 10 percent or above were up to four times as likely to have babies with birth defects.) Some endos who specialize in pregnancy might suggest you get your A1c under 6 percent, which is an average glucose reading of 126 mg/dL or lower. Nondiabetic A1cs, for comparison, are 4 to 6 percent, which is 68 to 126 mg/dL.

How do you bring those numbers down, living with a condition that's defined by high blood sugars? This was my biggest concern as a longtime diabetic who'd seen blood sugars range between 40 and 400 mg/dL in a single day. The answer is ongoing, regular blood sugar tests, up to 12 to 15 times a day. This means testing before meals, one hour and two hours after each meal, before bed, before and during exercise, during the night, and anytime you feel you might be having a low or just want to see where things are at.

"The blood sugar level targets for pregnancy seem unachievable when considering becoming pregnant, but it's totally doable," said Meredith Carroll, 39, type 1, from the Boston, Massachusetts, area and the mother of two kids aged 4 and 6. "As you increase the number of blood sugar tests per day, A1cs seem to come down on their own because you're on top of it. I saw excellent results in terms of my A1cs almost immediately, so it wasn't hard to maintain the changes."

Can your numbers ever be too low?[4] Brief episodes of hypoglycemia (low blood sugars) do not hurt the baby within. However, in addition to the unpleasant feeling of frequently being low and the importance of waiting to drive until your blood sugar is in a normal range, fetal growth might be restricted if your average blood sugars are around 86 mg/dL, or with an A1c of 4.6 percent or lower. According to research published in the *American Journal of Obstetrics and Gynecology* in 1990 that looked only at gestational diabetics (i.e., those who developed diabetes only during pregnancy), women whose average blood sugars were 86 mg/dL or lower had a higher risk of delivering babies who were small for their gestational age. Talk to your doctor if you find your A1cs are at or approaching this level.

Strategies for Maintaining Blood Sugars

Once you get into the habit of checking your blood sugar so often, it's likely to become second nature, even if you're checking at times that are new to you or when you'd rather be doing something else, like sleeping through the night. "Test, test, and test," said Carol Speight, 39, from Fleet, Hampshire, United Kingdom, whose daughter is 5. "You catch the inevitable highs and lows during pregnancy quicker and avoid possible problems. I tested at least twice a night during the whole of my pregnancy." Testing in the middle of the night can help you catch blood sugars so low that your liver kicks in and causes what's called a rebound high or the Somogyi effect. This high occurs when blood sugars go really low (which, if you're sleeping, you might not notice) and the body releases hormones that help raise the sugars quickly so that your brain can still function. Such highs are often tough to bring down, so avoiding them by treating lows in the middle of the night can help keep everything in line. This may mean setting your alarm clock for 3 a.m., but check what your doctor wants you to do before you start interrupting a good night's sleep every single night. Then again, think of it as practice for newborn feeding schedules.

To test your sugars, you'll need a blood glucose meter, test strips, a lancet, and, if you like, a spring-loaded device that will lance your finger at the push of a button. (I call mine my "finger-pricker"; your name for the device may be different.) I bring my meter everywhere with me: it's on the bedside table during the night, in my purse throughout the day, and on the elliptical trainer in the water bottle holder when I hit the gym. I use only one meter because I like to check my average readings and because I'd lose the extras. You may prefer to keep several meters in different places, at work and at home, or wherever. Meters are typically inexpensive; look for freebies at your doctor's office or promotions when companies introduce new models. If you can't find free ones, insurance often covers the cost. However, it's the test strip costs that bleed people with diabetes (or their insurance companies) dry. If having more than one meter helps you test more often, more power to you; just make sure you're well stocked up on the accompanying strips.

With all this close monitoring and subsequent correcting, you're bound to have more low blood sugar reactions (also known as hypoglycemia or insulin reactions). These let you know they're occurring because you can feel sluggish, jittery, hungry, cranky, sweaty, drained, or just not yourself. It's like an unwanted visit from the Hypo Seven Dwarves. Living so close to the normal range means your sugars don't have far to fall before you're having lows. Carrying a fast-acting simple sugar in your meter can help you treat these reactions as soon as you notice them. I carry LifeSavers because they fit into my glucose meter and are easy and relatively inexpensive to replace. You may prefer to drink juice or carry glucose tablets or have your own method of battling lows. The trick with treating these reactions, particularly if they're quite low, is fighting the urge to eat the entire refrigerator. The standard treatment for a low is to eat only 15 grams of fast-acting carb (which is five to six LifeSavers, four to six ounces of fruit juice, or three to four glucose tablets), wait out the low for 15 minutes, and see whether you're back in normal range. If you're not, chow another 15 grams of carb and wait another 15.

As someone who once ate four packs of LifeSavers to bring up my sugars and who used to eat Reese's Peanut Butter Cups to treat lows (because I couldn't eat them the rest of the time), let me tell you that the 15–15 rule, as it's called, is annoying and can feel like an eternity when you're suffering through the eggshell-knees, sweat-filled, heart-racing feeling of a low. However, it usually works and has prevented me from spiraling up from a 60 mg/dL blood sugar to 240 mg/dL within an hour. Treating by the rule generally brings my blood sugar up to around 90 mg/dL if I'm patient and just wait it out. Muddling around with peanut butter cups or, another favorite, globs of peanut butter straight from the jar complicates things because the high fat content blunts the absorption of the simple carb into your bloodstream, so it takes longer for your blood sugar to rise. It can also cause you to go high hours later, making for an unpleasant few hours of correcting highs and responding to lows, back and forth.

Technology Talk

Of course, testing all the time won't help your blood sugars stay in range unless you're also correcting for any high numbers with an extra hit of insulin. The amount you take is determined by your correction factor, or how many points your blood sugar will drop when you take one unit of insulin to bring down a high number. To get this insulin in you, you use an insulin pump or you take multiple daily insulin injections. For type 1 women, taking insulin is probably old hat by now. For those with type 2, being told you have to start on insulin might be no big deal, or it might freak you out.

Injecting Insulin

As mentioned earlier, most women with type 2 diabetes start taking insulin so that they can stay within the recommended pre-pregnancy and pregnancy range. Jennifer Grizzle, now 44, had taken pills to treat her type 2 for four years before she decided to try to get pregnant. Her doctor counseled her to take insulin as soon as she started trying to conceive.

"As a child and even as an adult, I have had a shaky relationship with needles," she said. "I don't like to see a needle coming towards me. I was sweating bullets with that first shot."

A nurse tried to reassure Grizzle by showing her how small the needle was and helped her pinch a fold of her thigh as she quickly pushed the needle into her skin.

"I had tears in my eyes, but I quickly realized it didn't hurt," Grizzle recalled. "Okay, I can do this," she thought. She began taking four shots a day, and with each one she'd repeat to herself, "You're doing this for a perfect baby." Her daughters, born healthy, are now 12 and 14.

If you think you could never become a human pincushion, you're not alone and you're not the first woman with diabetes to feel this way. It does get easier, often sooner than you might anticipate. Here are some tips on taking insulin for the first time:

- Pick an injection spot that works for you. If you can't or don't want to reach around to poke yourself in the ass, don't. Any fleshy part of the body will do, but typically the arms, thighs, hips, butt, or belly are recommended. You do need to rotate your sites, and you want to stay away from body parts that might not have a lot of subcutaneous fat, such as your calves or forearms. You may curse it the rest of the time, but when you are giving yourself shots, fat is your friend. And if you want to use an arm, stand in a doorway or sit on a chair with a tall back; propping your arm against the door frame or the chair back will mimic the action of pinching a fold of flesh on that upper-arm area—without needing a third hand.

- There are nerve endings everywhere underneath your skin, and one area might be particularly sensitive while another feels okay. Resting the edge of the needle lightly against your skin before you inject can help you find a spot that hurts less than another area.

- Pinch a pad of fat. This will help you avoid injecting into any muscle underneath the fat below your skin.

- I was taught to inject a needle quickly, like throwing a dart. I've never done that: it freaks me out too much. Instead, I slowly push the needle against my skin at a 90-degree angle until it breaks the surface and goes in smoothly. Sort of like an Olympic diver.

- There are automatic injectors that will do the dirty work for you, but in my opinion it's just as easy to learn to give yourself a shot manually. Parenthood will be full of explosive diaper blowouts and cleaning vomit off your shoulder and the hallway rug. What's one more unpleasantry to deal with? At least when you give yourself a shot, you can control when and how it happens. Being yakked on? Not so much.

Insulin Pumps

Insulin pumps are common these days, and if you're not already using one, going on one will, in my opinion, make it much easier to manage your pregnancy and your diabetes. I've been on a pump for nearly a decade and I'm biased, so don't just listen to me.

"Five years ago, I went on an insulin pump knowing in the back of my mind that someday I would want to have kids and would need to have my sugars in as close to perfect control as possible," said Randi Schwartz Carr, 31, type 1, of Iowa. Her daughter is now 2½. Randi was able to lower her A1c dramatically while on the pump, from a high of 11.9 percent the day she started the pump to 7.6 percent a month later, and she says she's been able to maintain A1cs in the upper 5 percent to lower 6 percent range, with a lot of work. While the pump is not magic, it is a tool that you can use, along with a lot of blood sugar testing, carbohydrate counting, stress management, and exercise, to get your A1c numbers within range. The advantages of being on a pump are that you can take smaller amounts of insulin than you can with a syringe and that you aren't poking yourself more than once just to deliver insulin. Some people believe that the basal infusion of insulin (a small amount of insulin going into the body all day long) mimics a working pancreas more closely than does a shot of long-acting insulin such as NPH. Varying the basal rate throughout the day allows you to fine-tune your insulin levels, which is tougher to do with multiple injections.

Going on an insulin pump is a major decision, and some women have compared it to being diagnosed with diabetes all over again. Pump trainers will work with you to ensure you understand exactly how the pump works. They'll also help you learn how to deal with problems such as clogs or malfunctioning infusion sets (the part that sits on your skin and lets the insulin enter your body subcutaneously). These problems can cause diabetic ketoacidosis, which occurs when the body does not have enough insulin to convert food into nutrients and acids build up in the blood. Trainers teach new pumpers about the necessity of testing blood sugar regularly and correcting high or low blood sugars immediately. There are also the emotional aspects of going on a pump and feeling connected to a piece of machinery all the time, and the practical consideration of where to place the pump during sleep or sex or even just when you are wearing a tight dress. Several resources that discuss choosing an insulin pump and using it effectively are available; see the Resources section at the end of this book for a list of books and websites.

Multiple Daily Injections

Some women remain on multiple daily injections instead of pumping for a number of reasons, including financial constraints, insurance coverage, plastic allergies, and a dislike of being attached to an insulin pump. Lisa, 29, type 1, from Canada, is currently trying to conceive. She takes a minimum of 5 injections each day, and may take up to 10 shots if she needs to correct a high number between meals or at bedtime. "I am just now approaching my target A1c of less than 7, after being 7.8 four months ago," she said. Financially, it makes more sense for her to choose multiple daily injections instead of an insulin pump, even though her blood sugars are higher than where she wants them to be, she said. "I have always been higher than the recommended values, so although many people out there do a better job, I'm happy I'm moving in the right direction."

Although there are different types of insulin available (fast acting versus longer acting) and complementary medications such as Symlin can help prevent postmeal blood sugar spikes, your doctor may hesitate to let you continue taking a newer medication like Symlin or Lantus (a long-acting insulin) because it hasn't been specifically or extensively studied in a pregnant population. (But see the Notes section for two small studies that found Lantus to be well tolerated during pregnancy.)[5] Instead, your doc may suggest that you switch to NPH, an insulin that's been available for longer, or that you forgo starting or staying on Symlin altogether. Talk to your doctor about which insulins and other medications are recommended during pregnancy, and if you are told to switch to something you're not used to, keep an eye out for any unexplained fluctuations in your blood sugars or other changes.

Continuous Glucose Monitors

CGMs have been available for some time, but U.S. insurance companies are only slowly coming around to covering them in the same way as insulin pumps, test strips, and other medical supplies. CGMs give you ongoing data from a sensor inserted under the skin to measure blood sugar readings minute by minute. They can show you trends, such as whether your blood sugar is increasing, decreasing, or holding steady. The CGM system isn't foolproof; you still need to calibrate it by doing a few fingersticks each day with a traditional glucose meter and entering the data into the CGM. However, at any given time, a CGM can provide an approximation of where your blood sugar is and where it is headed in a way that multiple daily fingersticks just can't match.

"I decided to use a CGM to help me work towards a lower A1c, and that was absolutely in pursuit of a healthy pregnancy," said Kerri Morrone Sparling, 30, type 1, of Rhode Island. She is 30 weeks pregnant. "Since my numbers have always been tough to control, I wanted all the technological help I could get. Seeing the constant feedback from my CGM has helped me respond to trends and stay on top of my diabetes."

When you are pregnant, the CGM can really help with keeping numbers in line. "I asked my perinatologist at the beginning of my pregnancy if I could get the CGM, but it did not arrive until my second trimester," said Sara Bancroft, 27, type 1, of Liverpool, New York, whose son is 1 and was born healthy. "Up until that point, my A1c was steady in the upper 5s, but after using the CGM, I was able to achieve my lowest A1c in 21 years of living with diabetes: 4.5! I think the key was being able to catch high numbers on the way up, before they became a problem. I called it 'actively correcting' my blood sugars in real time. It was also very helpful in the postpartum period to be able to find a basal that worked for me. I look forward to using my CGM for the full 40 weeks in future pregnancies! I truly attribute my son's health to being able to have such tight control over my blood sugars during pregnancy."

There are a few considerations, though. Like starting on an insulin pump, wearing a CGM means you have another medical device hanging on your waistband (unless you choose a model that is packaged with an insulin pump). Sometimes the numbers are inaccurate, and it's yet another machine that is subject to wear and tear—for which you'll be responsible. And, if your insurance company won't cover the costs, life with the monitor can be pricey if you're paying out of pocket for the main device or the sensors (the part that is inserted into the skin and transmits readings to the main device).

However, for pre-pregnancy and pregnancy blood sugar control, the CGM can be very helpful. It can be "a terrific tool that can help rein in hard-to-manage numbers," said Sparling. "It's not a miraculous machine that makes diabetes easy, but it does give me an edge."

What to Eat When You're Planning to Get Pregnant

You can probably guess that eating right will help ensure that your baby gets all the nutrition it needs in utero, but starting to eat well (or maintaining your already healthy habits) before pregnancy is also key. Taking a prenatal vitamin will ensure you're getting everything you need nutritionally and will give you enough folic acid to help protect against birth defects such as spina bifida. Food is covered in more detail in Chapter 3, but the quick specifics are here.

Counting carbohydrates helps you know how what you're eating will affect your blood sugars. The carbohydrate content of foods typically is measured in grams (and are also called carbs or carb, for short). A slice of white bread is 15 grams of carbohydrates, a glass of skim milk is 12 grams, and a 2.17-ounce bag of Skittles tropical flavor candies is 56 grams. Depending on your insulin-to-carb ratio, you can tailor the dose of insulin you take for a meal to how many carbs are in the meal. If your ratio were 1 unit of insulin to 10 grams of carbs, you'd take 1.5 units for the slice of bread, 1.2 units for the milk, and 5.6 units for the bag of candy.

Carbohydrate counting can also help you if you're not using insulin to treat your diabetes. Or you may be told to follow a food exchange system, where you're supposed to eat a certain number of servings of carbohydrates, proteins, and fats a day and are counseled on serving size and food choices. Talking with a nutritionist who is knowledgeable about diabetes and pregnancy can be helpful if these are new concepts for you.

Counting carbs is easy if you eat packaged foods; in the United States, the nutritional information is right on the side of the wrapper or box. But packaged food isn't the healthiest way to eat, and when you're eating for two, docs will tell you to eat nutrient-packed food so that your growing baby will get what it needs to thrive. (Sorry, Skittles.) And for women with diabetes, pregnancy shouldn't be the I-can-eat-anything-'cause-I'm-pregnant free-for-all carnival many nondiabetic women engage in. Sure, you're eating for two, but you need only an extra 300 calories of food a day (and typically those extra calories are required only in the second and third trimesters). Eating well before you're pregnant will help you stay on track while you're pregnant. Maintaining normal blood sugar levels is your top concern. Eating too much ensures extra weight that'll be that much harder to drop after the baby arrives—totally not your goal.

How do you carb count when the carb numbers aren't readily available? Many pocket-sized carbohydrate guides and several online databases will tell you the carb count of just about every food there is (see Resources). Many restaurants put nutritional information about their items online. If you're at a sandwich shop and you want to know how many carbs are in the bulkie roll, ask the behind-the-counter person whether you can take a look at the bread package.

People have different dietary strategies for maintaining blood sugars before and during pregnancy. Personally, I found it easier to eat the same breakfast and lunch nearly every day because I knew how my blood sugars would react. For breakfast, I'd eat pre-measured instant oatmeal, Splenda, and a dollop of peanut butter, with some grapes or raspberries thrown into the mix, plus I'd drink a glass of skim milk. The entire thing was healthy, delicious, and approximately 50 grams of carb. I could take the same amount of insulin each day and see predictable results one hour and two hours after the meal. Lunch was a grilled chicken sandwich with Swiss cheese, with a dab of herb mayo, onions, and cucumbers on whole-grain bread. It was relatively high in carbs, but again I knew what to take for it, which kept my sugars within range most of the day. Dinner was the wild card, but checking sugars after meals and through the night helped keep me on track. Eating this way for several months resulted in the best blood sugars and A1cs of my diabetic life, well within the target range for pregnancy with diabetes. And while I occasionally strayed from my breakfasts and lunch choices because, c'mon, that's a long time to eat exactly the same thing, I really enjoyed those two meals a lot. As a result, it rarely felt like I was depriving myself when I ate my glorious oatmeal, peanut butter, and grape concoction for breakfast instead of something else.

The Financial Realities of Pregnancy and Diabetes

Between the doctor's visits, the extra blood tests, the additional insulin, and maybe the expense of starting an insulin pump and/or a CGM, maintaining tight diabetes control while prepping for pregnancy and being pregnant is pretty darn spendy. And that's not even including all the gear, clothes, and furniture the baby will use once he or she is finally here. Although hand-me-down onesies or secondhand toys from yard sales and Craigslist can defray costs somewhat, there's no getting around the fact that supplies, appointments, and other things like parking and gas to get to those doc visits all add up.

If you're not independently wealthy from winning that multimillion-dollar lottery, planning ahead and saving can go a long way when you want your dollars to stretch. Putting aside money—under your mattress, in a regular savings account at your favorite bank, or in a health savings account through your (or your husband's or domestic partner's) job—can help you beef up your finances before your baby arrives. A health savings account allows you to take a portion of your (or your partner's) pretax salary and set it aside for medical expenses.

Usually, there are annual limits and the money must be used before the end of the calendar year. But, honestly, with diabetes there's always some appointment or supplies to fund. Just keep an eye on the paperwork necessary to get the money released directly to you from the health savings account so that you can pay the appropriate bill.

Health insurance in the United States can be an expensive, complex, and confusing topic, particularly if you (or your husband or partner) don't work for a company that automatically covers you simply for being an employee. For women with diabetes, having ongoing health insurance through an employer or a partner's employer is much easier (and potentially less expensive) than going without it and later trying to qualify for an individual policy after a gap in coverage. If you don't have health insurance before you get pregnant, look into the costs and the effort of buying an individual or family policy, and what it would take to qualify for group coverage through a school, alumni, professional, or trade association. While it's possible to get pregnant and maintain diabetes control without health insurance in the United States, it is an expensive (and potentially bankruptcy-triggering) proposition.

"We had spent time building up our savings, since the idea was that I would not go back to work and there was always the possibility of bed rest," said Anna Tang Norton, 34, type 1, of East Windsor, New Jersey. Her son is 19 months old. She and her husband had coverage for each other on their own insurance plans. "We had always used two insurances, both mine and my husband's, for years, as I found it was beneficial to have both for coverage on a new pump (I paid nothing for my last pump), prescriptions, pump supplies, and so on. It was wonderful when I gave birth; again, we paid for nothing—no ultrasounds, no doctor's visits, no additional testing, nothing at the hospital at birth. I'm glad we had coverage on both since I caught a glimpse of my hospital bill. Not including care for my son, it totaled over $80,000. This included four days in the hospital and all the expenses related to my c-section."

Scrutinize your existing health insurance policy so that you know exactly what is covered and what is expected to be an out-of-pocket expense. It's never a pleasure to get a shockingly high bill and to learn, long after the appointment, that it isn't covered by your insurance because of a rule you didn't know about beforehand. However, if you are pretty sure something should be covered and you receive a crazy high bill anyway, knowledge of your policy will give you more to work with when you call your insurance company to question the amount. And keep on top of annual changes that might affect your maternity, specialist, prescription, or durable medical equipment coverage, which often applies to insulin pumps and CGMs.

"I am very fortunate in the fact that finances were not a huge stress for me during my pregnancy," said Lindsay Gopin, 28, type 1, of Chicago, Illinois. Her daughter is 1 year old. "However, I did have to fight and advocate to get more test strips covered and get my continuous glucose sensor covered. I had to be very patient and persistent and eventually I was able to get what I needed."

Depending on where you live if you're outside the United States, you may still pay a considerable amount of money out of pocket if you want things that your plan doesn't cover. "I live in Canada and still find it expensive and eating up my savings," said Lisa. "My insurance doesn't cover testing supplies, pumps, newer types of insulin such as Lantus and Levemir, and only pays a portion of other insulins and other prescriptions."

Despite Everything: What to Do About Getting Pregnant With High Blood Sugars

What happens if you get pregnant before your A1c is where your doctor says it should be? Kassie, the author of the diabetes blog "noncompliant," knows that experience. She said her A1c was several points higher than the recommended range:

> My second pregnancy was unplanned. While I was taking steps to rein in my diabetes management, I wasn't there yet. It is so important to have your diabetes in great shape before you conceive. Women with diabetes should know that a normal or near-normal A1c reduces your baby's risk of birth defects to that of the nondiabetic population. When you conceive a baby with an out-of-range A1c, the risks loom disproportionately large and it's stressful. The first word out of my mouth when that second line appeared on the pregnancy test: "Shit." My endo's response, conveyed by a nurse: "Will you consider terminating?"

A planned pregnancy helps mitigate the worry that comes with conceiving with a high A1c. However, let me also say this: If you do get pregnant without being under 7 percent, and you wish to continue the pregnancy, understand that a high A1c doesn't guarantee problems, it just raises the risk.

Your response to any health care professional who berates you should be "Let's talk about how to do the best we can from here on out." Once my endo knew I was proceeding with the pregnancy, he and the CDE in his office were 100 percent on board with getting down to some serious diabetes work.

Risk Factors

If you have high blood sugars during pregnancy the chances of having a child with birth defects or other problems can be as high as 30 percent. This is 15 times the risk in the nondiabetic population. The general risk of birth defects with well-controlled sugars—the same as a nondiabetic's—is 2 percent. Another way to look at the risk of birth defects when sugars are uncontrolled is that even when your sugars are high, there is a 70 percent chance that your baby will not have any birth defects or other health problems. Of course, no one wants to put an unborn, wanted baby at risk for anything, so 3 chances out of 10 is still considerable. But, as Kassie says, if you are committed to continuing the pregnancy despite your less-than-optimal sugars at conception, talk seriously with your doctor about what you need to do to get your sugars within range throughout the rest of your pregnancy.

What actual risks are we talking about? The list includes defects of the spinal cord and the skeletal, urinary, reproductive, and digestive systems, heart problems, excess amniotic fluid, and the baby's size and weight.

The American Diabetes Association lists the chances of having a child with diabetes on the basis of genetic factors listed in the table on the next page.

Genetic disorders can occur in an otherwise healthy pregnancy with tight control. These include cystic fibrosis, sickle-cell disease, and Tay-Sachs. Genetic testing before you try to conceive will determine whether you are at risk for such conditions. If you are, you will be offered counseling to decide what to do with this information.

The Genetics of Diabetes: Your Child's Risk[6]

Neither parent has diabetes	1/11 chance of type 2 1/100 chance of type 1

Mother has type 1
    Child born before age 25
    Child born after age 25
	
	 1/25 chance of type 1
	 1/100 chance of type 1

Father has type 1	1/17 chance of type 1
Parent with type 1 by age 11	Child's risk of type 1 doubles
Both parents have type 1	1/4 to 1/10 chance of type 1

One parent has type 2
    Before age 50
    After age 50
	
	 1/7 chance of type 2
	 1/13 chance of type 2

Both parents have type 2	About 1/2 chance of type 2

© 2009 American Diabetes Association. From http://www.diabetes.org. Modified with permission from The American Diabetes Association.

Your endo will also want to test to ensure that your body is able to handle the demands of pregnancy. Diabetes can affect your eyes, heart, kidneys, and nerves, and as pregnancy can influence or worsen any potential problems you are already facing. Because of this, you may be asked to discontinue certain medications (an angiotensin-converting enzyme inhibitor for prevention of kidney issues, for example, or a statin for cholesterol control) because they aren't good for the developing baby, even though they are probably keeping your own health problems at bay. You may be asked to see additional specialists, such as an eye doctor to determine how your retinas look and whether you may need laser treatment before or during pregnancy to ensure your eye health is top-notch. Talk to your doc about what might affect you specifically, given your health history. Typical pre-pregnancy tests include screenings for your kidneys, eyes, blood pressure, thyroid hormone and cholesterol/triglyceride levels, peripheral neuropathy (nerve damage), depression, stress, and anxiety.

Finally, a good endo should also tell you that tight diabetes management is measured in your long-term blood sugar control. High blood sugars will happen—we have diabetes and, frankly, that's what the condition is all about—but the occasional high shouldn't cause lasting damage to your kid. With constant blood sugar testing, careful insulin corrections to bring sugars down, and measured amounts of handy, fast-acting sugar to bring you out of lows, your A1cs are likely to get where you want them to be.

Having a healthy pregnancy with diabetes is a lot of work, but consider it a solid foundation for the next stretch of the road. Whether your journey to seeing the double lines of a positive pregnancy test is simple or challenging, get ready for the next step of the way: your first trimester.

The First Trimester:
Grace Under Pressure

2

I See Two Lines—Now What?

Congratulations—you're pregnant! Is your mind racing? Tuck any thoughts about what could go wrong into the back of your head, and focus on what you're doing, why you're doing it, and how great it is (and will be). People will try to give you tons of advice, and some of it will be useful, but some of it will be pretty outdated—or simply wrong—when it comes to diabetes and pregnancy. This applies to everyone: your health care providers, your family, your friends, and especially those pesky people who always seem to have something negative to say. Knowing the facts about your own health will keep you confident and in charge of your pregnancy and your body.

Enjoy the Moment

For some women, this may be ridiculous advice. Of course you're enjoying the moment. There's all sorts of stuff to do, like onesies to ogle and bigger boobs to flaunt. For the rest of us, though, this may be when the worrying kicks up even more. How can you enjoy the moment when you're wondering what your damn blood sugar is All The Time? Even if you have a CGM attached to your belly (and, if so, will you need to find a new place for it?) or you just prick your fingers and test yourself all day and night (and even if you don't), those blood sugars are going to be the bane of the next nine or so months. Aren't they?

Well, yes and no.

Michelle Kowalski, now 34, of Phoenix, Arizona, found out she was pregnant with her third child at 30—just two months after being misdiagnosed with prediabetes (a precursor to developing type 2 diabetes). "I freaked out because I knew very little about diabetes and pregnancy, and when I did Internet research, all I found were horror stories," she recalled. "I was afraid to eat anything." Her A1c was 7 percent, which she described as being "not terrible, but not the greatest." She met with a CDE, who told her she most likely had type 2 diabetes and not prediabetes. Kowalski immediately began injecting a long-acting insulin and started to keep records of her blood sugars, food intake, and exercise routines. Her CDE "encouraged me with literally everything. She went over my logs and offered advice based on what she saw." With such support, Kowalski became diligent about what and when she ate, which led to better blood sugar control. Her CDE helped her "realize that the horror stories are just horror stories and that as long as I kept eating right, exercising, testing my blood sugar, keeping in touch and taking her advice, I would have a healthy happy pregnancy and a healthy happy baby." Her youngest daughter was born without any health problems.

Finding out you are pregnant unexpectedly can be tough and can affect your sugars in the short term (even if your long-term blood sugars are in good shape). Keep an eye on the numbers and do what you can to correct highs as soon as possible. "I didn't plan on getting pregnant, so it was stressful when I found out," said Traicy Lewis, 33, type 1, of Finleyville, Pennsylvania. "I was not married and I wanted to be when I had a baby, and neither me nor the father had much money." Despite the challenges, Lewis's blood sugars stayed stable, much to her surprise. Her A1c was 5.9 percent at conception, and she worked hard to maintain tight blood sugars overall by carefully adjusting her insulin and listening to her doctors' suggestions. "I waited until I saw three days of high readings before I made an insulin adjustment," she said. "This let me know that it wasn't something else causing my sugar to rise, such as mild stress, hormones, underbolusing [taking too little insulin to cover a meal or snack], air bubbles in pump tubing, and so on." Such informed decisions can help you keep your blood sugars, and long-term A1c levels, within range.

Don't Freak Out

Knowledge is power, and that can give you confidence. The more you know about the realities of your particular pregnancy with diabetes—not some fuzzy ideas about the general concept—the better

you'll be able to reassure both yourself and others about any potential problems. That confidence, to be able to explain intelligently why
you are healthy and how your future kid has every chance of being
born healthy and awesome, is an excellent way to defuse some well-
intentioned soul who just wants to tell you about potential complications, birth defects, or some other horror-show idea that might never
apply to you at all.

This can be difficult to remember if you're sitting in a doctor's
office hearing about what could go wrong.

"I saw a high-risk obstetrician [before conceiving] and he gave
me a long speech about diabetes and risks, and the likelihood of
diabetes-related problems for the baby," said Carlynn, 34, type 1, of
Switzerland. "I was *extremely* upset and cried for about 10 minutes
in the hospital toilets before gathering myself enough to go home.
Afterwards, I was furious. I had had diabetes for three years at that
stage, and my A1c numbers were fine. My endocrinologist was happy
with me. I think it is vital to be prepared for this sort of response from
medical personnel—be prepared for medical staff to tell you horror
stories and assume you know nothing."

Because Carlynn immediately contacted her own endocrinologist
to discuss what the obstetrician had told her, she soon confirmed a
more realistic portrait of the health risks, based on her specific history. "The advantage of getting a second opinion is that you will have
calmed down, and you can see if the first doctor was simply a scare-
monger, or if some of his information needs to be taken into account,"
she said. "You'll get more information, and that is always useful."

Self-knowledge, too, can go a long way. Lindsay Gopin worked hard
to keep her A1cs within a tight range before conception. "I kept telling
myself to trust my body," she said. "If my body allowed me to get pregnant, then it would be able to make a healthy baby." At the same time,
she noted, she was extremely self-motivated to aim for and maintain
tight blood sugar control, both before and during her pregnancy. "The
fear is what drove me to be so successful in the journey," she said.

Of course, the journey is easier if you don't feel you're all alone.
Other women with diabetes who are pregnant can share insights about
such things as whether you can continue to use your abdomen as a
site for injections or infusion sets. (I did, right until the day I delivered; another friend told me her doctor nixed the idea until the baby's
arrival. Neither of us knows why the other's doctor advised what she

did, but at least we could discuss our experiences.) "Even though I treasured my CDE, it was often easier to hear the same thing from a diabetic mommy who had already been through what I was going through," said Michelle Kowalski. "I found an online support group where I could ask questions and get advice from people who were in the same boat as I was." (See the Resources section at the end of this book for online and other resources specifically for women with diabetes who are considering pregnancy or are already pregnant.)

Handling High Sugars, Past and Present

What's done is done, and while you may be someone who stresses about last week's high readings or this morning's rebound (a very low blood sugar level followed by a sky-high one), there ain't much that can be done about them now. The motto I live by, whether pregnant or not, is simply to test, correct, and move on. Others agree.

"I just took one day at a time," said Katrina Holm, 30, type 1, from Missouri City, Texas, who has two toddler girls. "It caused me more stress to wonder if that 300 mg/dL I saw on my meter caused damage to my baby than to just treat it, try to figure out what caused it, and try to correct it in the future."

Regularity during pregnancy covers more than simply your bathroom habits. If you tend to eat the same things, exercise at the same time, or generally have the same routine each day, it can be easier to pinpoint why your blood sugars show unexplained highs or a general trend upward. Also, ongoing testing, even if you're on a CGM, can help you catch and correct high blood sugars early. Sure, it's hardly reassuring to see that your blood sugar is 250 mg/dL, or even 150 mg/dL, but there's less potential for damage if it's only been an hour or two since you last took insulin. If you've been high for many hours or even many days, there's a bigger window of opportunity for a problem to develop.

If you're on multiple daily injections or use an older model of insulin pump, remember that you might have insulin working in your body when you test and see a high blood sugar reading. Rapid-acting insulins such as Humalog and NovoLog usually start working within 15 minutes, peak just before 2 hours, and are gone from the body about 6 hours later. So if you test 1 hour after a meal and are outside your target range, taking more insulin might send your blood sugar plummeting a few hours later. Using the "insulin on board" feature on most insulin pump models, or self-calculating how much insulin is working in your body by knowing when your insulin peaks, how long it lasts, and when you last took some, can help prevent crushing lows.

"I used [my insulin pump] to guide me as to how much insulin I needed according to the insulin sensitivity factor preset by my endocrinologist," said Josée Renaud, 24, type 1, of northern Ontario, Canada. She is midway through her first pregnancy. "I learned, while using a CGM, it can take up to several hours for the blood sugar to come back down to a normal range. You must be careful not to over-bolus and end up in a severe low due to excess insulin."

Exercise is another way to help bring down highs or maintain steady sugars, but it can take a lot of trial and error to figure out how it works best for you. Work out too hard and you might bottom out and need to gulp box after box of juice. Work out when your sugar is too high and the adrenaline kick you get might send your numbers even higher. The guideline for people with diabetes is to avoid exercise when their readings are above 250 mg/dL with ketones or above 300 mg/dL otherwise; if you're in the 200s and don't have any ketones, you might find that taking a small amount of insulin before exercising helps your sugars go down better than if you exercise without the insulin adjustment (See Chapter 5 for more specifics).

"I used exercise *a lot* to help with high blood sugars," said Lindsay Gopin. "If my sugar was about 150 mg/dL, I would give a small bolus and then go work out for 20 minutes to bring my sugar down quickly." Gopin, who works as a social worker in private practice and as a fitness trainer, cut back on work while she was pregnant so that she could maintain tight diabetes control; her A1cs ranged from 4.4 to 5.2 percent during that time. "I would exercise to bring down high blood sugars even at 3 a.m.," she said. "I have a treadmill and an elliptical trainer at home, and I would put on my sneakers without socks, get on the machine with my big belly, and just go."

Will I Grow a Fat Baby? Will My Kid Have Diabetes?

It's so commonly heard that it's practically a cliché: women with diabetes have big babies. Officially, it's called macrosomia, a term that refers to babies born around the 90th percentile for weight. With diabetes in the mix, the pregnant woman's body regularly deals with blood sugars that are higher than normal. All babies in utero receive the nutrients they need to grow directly from the mom's blood. Along with vitamins and nutrients, any extra glucose floating around moves over to your fetus's body. When the baby is developing normally, its pancreas senses the extra sugar infusion and secretes more insulin to keep its own blood sugar stable. This process packs more weight onto the developing baby's frame and can lead to macrosomia.

Of course, fat babies aren't guaranteed to moms with diabetes. As always, keeping your sugars under tight control means there's less glucose floating around for your babe to process. And big babies aren't always caused by diabetes, either. Maybe you and your husband are full-figured types and you both come from similarly built families. In this case, it's unlikely your newborn will weigh in at the lower end of the scale. Anything is possible, but don't discount the role your genes (in addition to the ones that may have contributed to a diabetes diagnosis) can have.

The genetics of diabetes was discussed in Chapter 1, but how do you handle knowing that the risks exist at all? On one hand, there's a relatively small chance your child will develop diabetes. There's a little risk of being hit by lightning, too. On the other hand, didn't lightning already strike when you were diagnosed with diabetes? Overall though, pregnancy and parenting are about knowing the potential risks of anything and being able to raise your child or children despite them. If the risks were truly going to ruin your quality of life, you probably would have avoided getting (or staying) pregnant in the first place.

My concerns about our son, Ethan, developing diabetes were most intense just after he was born. Despite my attempts to nurse, Ethan lost more than 10 percent of his body weight. When he was 3 days old, a nurse told me Ethan needed to start drinking formula to gain weight. I was disappointed because I had heard there was a potential connection between drinking formula made from cow's milk and developing diabetes. (Most commercial formula contains intact cow's milk proteins.) Nursing is also linked to a host of health benefits, among them a potential link to diabetes prevention. As a result, I insisted that Ethan drink a predigested formula that would be as delicate on his system as any formula could be, one that was being used in an ongoing research study of infants of type 1 mothers. (It was also much more expensive than a can of "regular" formula.) Nursing never worked for me, and

Ethan thrived with formula, but I continued to try to feed him breast milk. I pumped it around the clock for nearly nine months—as long as my meager supply held out. I also waited to give him any milk products until he was at least a year old, when his pediatrician assured me that the benefits of dairy consumption were greater than the still unproven risk that he might develop diabetes from consuming cow's milk as a toddler. (At the time, I couldn't find conclusive evidence to prove otherwise.)

I keep a container of Ketostix in Ethan's diaper changing area. These are over-the-counter strips that detect ketones in the urine. Ketones are a sign of very high blood sugar levels. Whenever he has a particularly wet diaper, I press a strip into the soaked fabric and watch to see whether the strip changes color, indicating the presence of ketones. So far, the strip color hasn't changed. I'd rather do that occasionally than prick his body to obtain a drop of blood, which I did once when I thought his breath smelled fruity (another sign of ketones). I cried as I prepared to stick Ethan's heel (he was only a few months old at the time, and blood is typically taken from the heel instead of the fingertip at that age). Seeing my distress, he began crying, too. I lanced his tiny heel, and I felt awful. Ethan's blood sugar was normal—and I was so relieved I promised myself I won't stick him again unless he requests it when he gets older or shows obvious signs of undiagnosed diabetes such as severe weight loss or excessive thirst. (And even then I'll probably have his doctor's office prick his finger; it's worth the $20 office co-payment to avoid the trauma of hurting him unnecessarily.)

My worries have subsided somewhat since my son's baby days. However, I tell myself that if my son ever does develop diabetes, he'll at least have a strong advocate and comrade with me as his mom. We'll be in it together.

As our kids grow up, such fears may wane because there are more pressing day-to-day things to deal with. "I think that I will always have a little worry in the back of my mind about it, but I do not think about it much," said Abby Nagel, 44, type 1, of Maplewood, New Jersey, whose two daughters are 6 and 3.

Others feel that the more they know, the more there is to anticipate. "I don't remember being worried while I was pregnant about my children developing diabetes, but I worry about it now," said Michelle Kowalski. "Now that I have four years of this under my belt and read what parents of children with diabetes go through, and knowing what

I go through, I constantly say I'm glad it's me who has diabetes and not my children."

Advocacy: Speaking Up for Yourself and Your Child

I don't know about you, but living with diabetes has made me a pushy broad. (Well, that and having a family who encouraged such behavior.) Diabetes has forced me to listen to my body and to puncture my fingers many times a day to check where my blood sugar is at, to heed the numbers if they're too high and exercise or take a smidge of insulin if I need to, and to pay attention to the signs of a low blood sugar even if I am doing something far more interesting. It means I sometimes need to drink juice even if I just brushed my teeth and the citrus flavor against the minty freshness of the toothpaste tastes awful. Diabetes helps me to ask many questions when I need to know how something might be affecting my body. (Is that twinge just a twinge, or is it the onset of permanent nerve damage in my thigh? Will laser eye treatment ruin my vision forever or allow me to keep reading and writing without assistance?) It also helps me ask questions when I need to know how something might be affecting my pocketbook. (Don't get me started on how many times I have called an insurance company to ask exactly why my bill looks the way it does.) The point of this is to encourage you to be an advocate, both for yourself as a pregnant woman with diabetes and for the person currently residing in your uterus. Maybe you're more Shrinking Violet than Squeaky Wheel, but the more confident and aware you are about what you and your kid-to-be need, and need to know, the more likely you are to ask the right questions, collect the right information, and demand the best care from your medical providers.

Who to Tell First and Where to Get Support

Being both a lifelong worrier and a bit superstitious, I held off revealing my pregnancy to anyone in person other than my husband and doctors until I was past my first trimester. I blogged anonymously about my experience of getting pregnant and posted developments as they happened, so my blog readers learned right away. But since they weren't people I knew personally, and they didn't know my real name, I didn't care that they knew. The one close friend who knew my blog and saw me often in real life was sworn to secrecy about the news. I was too worried about a miscarriage or other problems to announce anything, because I knew I would be devastated if I had to tell people the pregnancy had ended too early. When I finally did come out of the closet at my office, at 20 weeks, it was a relief to explain why I regularly wore baggy sweaters and looked fatter than everyone else. (My work colleagues were mostly rail thin and fashion forward.) "Thank God," said one. "I had wondered what was going on with you, and no one was going to ask."

Others can't wait to share their news. "I told people right away that I was pregnant—no waiting," said Erin Argueta, 39, type 1, of Stamford, Connecticut. Her kids are now 10 and 13. "I was *so* excited. I don't keep secrets very well, and I chose to tell *everyone*. I knew I ran a risk, but I'm a person who likes support from friends and family. If something had gone wrong, I knew I'd want them to know and be there for me. Luckily, both pregnancies were success stories."

Picking and choosing who to tell has its advantages, too. "I immediately told my parents and mother-in-law, because I knew that without their support, it would be difficult," said Anna Tang Norton. "With the others, we waited until the first trimester was over."

Support—from family, friends, or friends who feel like family—helps when you're juggling the myriad tasks that accompany pregnancy with diabetes. Some partners define the meaning of the word. Having my husband, Dave, get out of a warm bed in the midnight hour to grab me some LifeSavers from our kitchen downstairs to help me treat a low blood sugar was, and is, terrific and much appreciated (pregnancy or not). He also took off a lot of time from his job to accompany me to most of my doctor's appointments and asked questions I forgot to ask. Such actions let you know that while you are the one testing sugars and taking insulin and counting carbs, you're not alone. It's a nice preview of what parenting a child together might be like.

"My husband was and still is my biggest support and partner in living with diabetes," said Abby Nagel. "He is very knowledgeable about how to handle my highs and lows, and when I could not reach my tush to put in a new pump infusion site, he did it for me."

Other partners show their support by acknowledging all you're handling. "I was incredibly diligent about what I was doing," said Michelle Kowalski. "My husband knew how seriously I was taking it, and he never judged or questioned. He trusted me and what I was doing to manage my blood sugar."

And while they might not experience the feeling of a plummeting blood sugar, partners can help you stay focused on life beyond the low. Lindsay Gopin used jellybeans to treat insulin reactions and learned that one bean would raise her blood sugar by 10 points. "My husband would sit with me while I was low and remind me to only eat four jellybeans, so I wouldn't overeat and go too high."

But spouses aren't the only source of support, which can be reassuring if your partner isn't available or giving you what you need. Family and friends can be sources of help and encouragement. "My mother made sure that I didn't miss an appointment," said Traicy Lewis. "Sometimes that was three times a week doing nonstress tests at the hospital, 45 minutes away. I didn't drive at the time so that was going out of her way to do something for me."

Support groups, either in person or online, can also be beneficial. "I would also advise talking to other diabetic mothers on the Internet or in real life if you can," said Carlynn. "They are going through the same thing as you and understand what no one else can." If you're lucky enough to have a posse of diabetic pals, all the better. "I was fortunate to have a group of women friends who all were diabetic and were or were just pregnant," said Abby Nagel. "It was a great experience to have friends who were dealing with all the pregnancy and diabetes issues I was. They could empathize and gave me good tips on how to deal with lows, frequent testing, crazy blood sugar numbers, and constantly faxing what I ate and what my sugar readings were to my endo."

Explaining Yourself and the *Steel Magnolias* Mindset

People will likely follow your lead when they hear that you are both a woman with child and a woman with diabetes. If you're confident and informed, you can easily explain yourself when people ask you questions or try to give you advice. For many people who aren't intimately familiar with the topics of diabetes and pregnancy, the play and film *Steel Magnolias* might be the only reference they have. The 1989 movie is arguably the most common pop culture reference about diabetes and pregnancy (at least until this masterpiece becomes a bestseller).

Steel Magnolias is based on the true story of a woman with long-term type 1 diabetes.[1] Shelby, played by Julia Roberts, is about to get married. Her mother, M'Lynn, played by Sally Field, worries about Shelby's health. Early in the story, M'Lynn rushes to give a sweaty and volatile Shelby orange juice after a particularly dramatic insulin reaction. Later, it's revealed that Shelby has kidney damage as a result of her diabetes and her doctors have told her she should not get pregnant; the stress on her kidneys could kill her. Declaring that she'd rather have "30 minutes of wonderful than a lifetime of nothing special," Shelby purposefully gets pregnant and gives birth to a healthy son. Three years later, however, her kidneys have indeed worsened. Shelby undergoes dialysis and, later, a kidney transplant from M'Lynn, but it's not enough. Her body ultimately rejects the new kidney, Shelby lapses into a coma while waiting for additional corrective surgery, and she dies.

Robert Harling, the playwright and screenwriter, wrote the story after his sister Susan died in 1986 at age 32 from complications from type 1 diabetes. It is key to point out that at the time, personal blood sugar monitors were a fairly recent invention, and insulin pumps, rapid-acting insulin, and CGMs were either uncommon or simply hadn't been invented. The concept of intensive diabetes management then was very different from what it is today.

Also, Shelby specifically defies medical advice and gets pregnant. While not every person with diabetes has kidney or other complications, some do. If you have kidney, eye, heart, or other complications that a pregnancy would worsen or significantly affect, it is crucial to talk to your medical team—your endocrinologist, your OB/GYN, and any other medical specialist who manages your care with this complication—and find out exactly how a pregnancy will affect your health. Work with your doctors, not in spite of them, to do all that you can to maintain great health before, during, and after a pregnancy, and know the risks you face if all medical opinions urge you to avoid pregnancy altogether.

Dealing With the Commentary

You and I know that having diabetes doesn't necessarily mean that you'll have a sick or big baby or that it's a death sentence. How do you deal with people who still think that way, perhaps stuck in the *Steel Magnolias* mindset?

"Try not to get defensive about comments that people might say regarding pregnancy and diabetes," said Katrina Holm. "Remember that they may have preconceived notions about pregnancy and diabetes and that your best option is to try to educate them. Let them know that with a good A1c, and proper management of your diabetes, you can have a very healthy baby."

Hammering home that you understand your health needs clearly usually conveys that you know what you are doing and that you are doing it just fine. "I explain to people that I am really healthy and doing everything I can to take care of myself and my baby," said Lindsay Gopin. "I show my insulin pump and sensor and explain how it helps me."

Sometimes the comments and concern are secondhand, which can catch you off guard and be even worse because you can't immediately address the issues with the person who brought them up. "I didn't hear many negative comments during my pregnancy—I had a very good support group," said Anna Tang Norton. "My mom, however, had a bunch of friends who were very worried, praying all the time, and never failed to mention how large babies are when moms have diabetes." Norton also heard many "stories about how I shouldn't be pregnant in the first place. Hearing those stories felt like a slap in the face for me, especially since I had been focusing on my health for so long for this reason," she said.

Given everything else on your daily to-do list, it's your decision how much energy to expend educating others. "I never shy away from talking about my diabetes, but I don't advertise it, either," said Traicy Lewis. "If it's brought up, I talk about it. How are people going to know about it if I don't talk about it? The misconceptions have to be put to rest somehow, so I think it's my obligation to talk about it. If I didn't, everyone would still think it's extremely difficult for diabetics to have babies, which is nonsense if you get the proper care and take care of yourself."

Others have a different view. "I try to educate people but sometimes you can only do so much," said Erin Argueta. "It's not worth it to get upset about other people's ignorance."

Paging Dr. Amazing

No matter what you think about doctors and other health care professionals, you'll be dealing with them a lot if you're doing a preplanned, closely monitored pregnancy. It's ideal if you love the docs you see, but that's not always going to be the case. When you've found the doctors you will see during this pregnancy, communication is key for everyone. It's ideal to have doctors who work together and regularly communicate with each other about, say, your changing insulin needs or the results of your prenatal screening tests. If that doesn't happen, just make sure you are aware of what each doc is doing and why. If your obstetrician has prescribed Zofran for excessive nausea, for example, does your endocrinologist know that your insulin needs might change because previously you haven't been able to keep anything down but now you might start, thanks to the medication? Does your eye doctor know you are pregnant and that your tightened blood sugars may make your vision worse? (Strange irony there, right?) If your docs aren't in close contact, fill them in on all your medical happenings each time you have an appointment.

Talking With All the Docs

At any point during your pregnancy, it's possible you could be seeing an obstetrician, an endocrinologist, a perinatologist, an eye doctor, a nutritionist, a CDE, and other health care people. The collection of appointments, personalities, and points of view can seem overwhelming. How do you keep it all together?

Personally, Dave and I are big note-takers. One or both of us were busy writing during each appointment, and I eventually filed and kept most of the information. It was a way to document the pregnancy, sure, but it was also a way to keep track of who said what and when. Maybe notes aren't your thing. Figure out a way to document progress or planned changes in your routine so that you can remember to make those changes and let the rest of your health care team know what's going on.

Even if you've dealt with diabetes for a long time, carrying a child is usually a new experience. You may have been pregnant before or have a boatload of kids by now, but every pregnancy is different. While you might know how your body responded the last time you were with child, there's often something that is novel.

"While you have your own knowledge about diabetes and how your body reacts in certain situations, remember that it can be refreshing to hear other points of view from experienced professionals," said Josée Renaud. "And just as there are good and bad people out there,

there are some professionals who have less understanding of life with diabetes, and others who have excellent knowledge and are anxious to help."

At the same time, speak up and ask if you don't understand something or if a suggestion sounds really out there. "Ask lots of questions [if you are told] what you 'need' to be doing," said Lindsay Gopin. "Ask why. My nutritionist told me I had to be eating *at least* 50 carbs per meal, and when I asked why, she didn't even really know. I followed a lower-carb diet while pregnant and I think this is what also helped me to control my sugars so well."

Your doctors and medical team should want to help you to have the healthiest pregnancy you can. They should be respectful if you are sincerely trying to keep your blood sugars in range and your eating habits in line. "I think you need to speak with them with an open mind. I find that it helps in the way the team treats you as a patient," said Anna Tang Norton. "I always have taken advice well and have tried to act on it. Sometimes I am successful, sometimes not." Managing blood sugars can be an art as well as a science, and the numbers sometimes fluctuate without a rational explanation. "Because of this, and the frustrations that go along with it, it's very important to work with a good, responsive, and up-to-date team of medical professionals," said Tang Norton.

How to Weigh All the Opinions and Be Your Own Advocate

With so many appointments and doctors, you'll hear a lot of medical advice and suggestions about what to do to be as healthy as possible, both for yourself and for your growing child. Will you follow every piece of advice without question? Some things, such as techniques for keeping your blood sugars in range, may make more sense than others, such as the well-meaning, but in my opinion unnecessary, admonishment to change your lancet every single time you prick your finger to test your blood sugar. It can be overwhelming to keep track of everything, from ensuring you have enough insulin and other supplies on hand, to having a glucose source ready if you go low, to managing all the appointments you have scheduled. What do you follow and what do you skip?

"I think it's a trial-and-error situation," said Anna Tang Norton. "For the last several years, I have worked with an endocrinologist who has approached my diabetes with me as a team. I ask questions and he answers. He asks me questions and I answer. Together, we come up with solutions and ideas on how to fix things."

Others push to know why something has been prescribed. "I did a lot of my own research," said Lindsay Gopin. "I would listen to what others suggested and research until I found out my own philosophy on an issue."

Gopin kept her sugars under extremely tight control and argued with her medical team about her desire to deliver her daughter whenever the baby was ready to arrive. (Women with diabetes are often counseled to deliver by around 38 weeks because of concerns about placental breakdown and potentially larger babies.) "I had to fight, literally, to tell my gynecologist that delivering at 38 weeks was ridiculous, because with my A1c, my baby was fine," she said. "My blood sugars are better than half your patients without diabetes," she told them. "I asked for more data, more research, to support their position, and all the data they showed me was from back in the 1970s."

No doubt reassured by her tight control, her doctors let Gopin progress to 41 weeks, but no longer. Had her obstetrician refused, Gopin said, she would have gotten a second opinion at the same hospital, a top-notch, highly respected medical center in Chicago. "I kept saying, 'Why treat me like a diabetic when my body is not acting like one?' Ironically, on the day I was scheduled for an induction, I went into natural labor," she said. After 36 hours of labor, her daughter was born healthy and at a normal weight. In Gopin's words, "doctors have never really helped me, because I do it all myself."

While you may not share such strong opinions, it is true that most doctors aren't living with diabetes the way you and I are. Something that works for a group of your doctor's patients with diabetes may not work for you, and vice versa. Being your own advocate means knowing what works for you, and your child, even if it goes against conventional wisdom.

"Being your own advocate is critical," said Lindsay Gopin. "It's an important skill to learn before you become a parent, too. You know that you know your body the best." Josée Renaud agrees. "I consider [medical advice and other people's opinions], but I never let them take over my own," she said. "Many people have absolutely no clue about what living with diabetes fully encompasses, and will never realize what it truly is in their lifetime."

3

What Do I Eat?

Eating while you're pregnant can be a challenge. Throw blood sugar control into the mix and you may wonder what the heck you're going to consume for the next nine months. Sashimi and soft cheese, for example, may have been great for your sugars because their lack of carbs helped things stay steady. But now such foods are usually considered off limits because of problems they can cause for a developing fetus. And what are you supposed to do about morning (or all-day) sickness? Here's how to eat and drink smartly for two, which will help your sugars stay in check, ensure your kid develops properly, and keep you from feeling deprived, hungry, or simply powerless in the face of your pregnancy cravings.

Nutrition for Any Pregnancy

Before you even get pregnant (because you're planning things in advance as I wrote about back in Chapter 1, right?), talk to your obstetrician about going on a stand-alone folic acid supplement or a prenatal vitamin that contains the recommended amount of folic acid. According to the March of Dimes, the leading nonprofit organization for pregnancy and baby health, taking at least 400 micrograms of folic acid (the synthetic form of folate, a B vitamin) daily is a proven way to help protect a baby from developing brain and spinal cord defects such as spina bifida in utero.[1] It's also a good idea to eat enough folate (the natural form of the vitamin) from foods such as fortified breakfast cereals and other enriched grains, orange juice, cooked broccoli, legumes such as black beans and lentils, and leafy green vegetables such as spinach.

A prenatal vitamin will help you round out some other nutritional needs you might be missing from your diet. (However, a prenatal vitamin won't provide *all* the nutrients you or your kid will need, so definitely plan to eat a well-balanced diet in addition to taking a pill.) It's key to eat really well during pregnancy so that your baby gets exactly what it needs to thrive. Your doctor may prescribe a specific prenatal vitamin, but over-the-counter varieties often have what you need as well. A solid prenatal includes vitamins A, B6, B12, C, D, E, and K, folic acid (usually at least 800 micrograms, if not 1,000 micrograms—ask your health care provider how much you should take), niacin, riboflavin, thiamin, calcium, iodine, iron, magnesium, phosphorus, and zinc.[2] Talk to your doctor about how much of each ingredient you should take in supplement form; some vitamins are toxic at high doses, while others are not.

Calcium is important for building both your baby's and your own teeth and bones.[3] Particularly in the second trimester, your baby needs calcium. If you don't get enough calcium in your diet, the baby will take what it needs from your skeleton; this deficit can lead to osteoporosis when you're older. It's recommended you get 1,000 milligrams of calcium each day. Calcium is found in dairy foods such as (low-fat or skim) milk, cheese, yogurt, tofu, broccoli, almonds, and enriched orange juice.

Beyond talking a prenatal vitamin, though, what exactly does eating well mean? Consuming a variety of foods such as fruits, vegetables, whole-grain breads and pastas, milk and other dairy products, beans, lean red meat, poultry, and fish that's low in mercury will ensure that you get the vitamins and nutrients you and your growing baby need.[4]

Each person is different, and it's best to choose a diet that is both healthful and tasty so that you'll enjoy and want to eat what you're eating each day. Some people, as I wrote in Chapter 1 and did myself, decide to eat the same or similar meals daily. In doing so, the carb counts and the effects of the food are well known, and the variables are minimized (provided you're eating enough nutrients and vitamins each day). Knowing exactly what you ate and how it affected you in the past makes it (somewhat) easier to fine-tune insulin doses to try to ensure future tight control. Eating different breakfasts for nine months and figuring out nine months' worth of different insulin doses involves a lot more mental effort than knowing you'll be eating a bowl of a half cup of oatmeal with a half cup of berries and a tablespoon of peanut butter and a glass of skim milk every morning and that the fat in the peanut butter will smooth out the numbers after breakfast and keep you from feeling hungry too soon afterward. This is particularly helpful once your insulin ratios start changing (around weeks 19 through 26 in the second trimester).

"We try to individualize dietary advice," said Emmy Suhl, MS, RD, CDE, of the Joslin Diabetes Center's Nutrition and Diabetes Education program in Boston, Massachusetts. "Our overarching aims are to help pregnant women achieve their target blood glucose goals and, at the same time, eat healthfully. The healthful eating goal allows for considerable latitude in food choices." The Joslin Diabetes Center also follows recommendations from the Institute of Medicine, a nonprofit organization that gives science-based health advice and is an arm of the National Academy of Sciences.[5] The institute calls for a minimum carbohydrate intake of about 135 grams of carbs a day for pregnant women, said Suhl (up to 175 grams daily, with 28 grams of fiber considered an adequate daily amount; carbs are found in varying quantities in sugars, grains, cereals, pasta, legumes, fruits, some dairy foods, and some vegetables, particularly starchy ones). Suhl advises lower-carb diets for people who can't meet their blood sugar targets while eating that amount of carbs; this is more commonly seen in those with type 2 diabetes than in those with type 1. The Institute of Medicine also recommends eating 70 grams of protein and 27 milligrams of iron, and it considers 20–35 grams of fat daily an acceptable amount for proper nutritional needs.

Suhl noted that the American Diabetes Association recommends avoiding saturated fat and trans fats in favor of monounsaturated and polyunsaturated fats.[6] Saturated fats and trans fats are currently believed to raise cholesterol levels, while mono- and polyunsaturated fats are currently believed to help lower them. Foods high in saturated fats include full-fat dairy foods such as cheese, butter, regular ice cream, and whole and 2 percent milk, meats such as beef, veal, lamb, and pork, lard, the skin of chicken or turkey, coconut, and items made with coconut, palm, or palm kernel oils. Foods with trans fats include processed foods such as French fries, doughnuts, cookies, crackers, muffins, pies, and cakes made with hydrogenated or partially hydrogenated oils, stick margarines, or shortening. Monounsaturated and polyunsaturated fats are found in plant-based foods such as avocados, canola, olives, olive/peanut/safflower/soybean/sunflower oils, walnuts, almonds, peanuts, peanut butter, pumpkin/sesame/sunflower seeds, and some soft (tub) margarines, as well as in fish such as salmon and trout. It's also a good idea to choose low-fat or skim versions of milk, cheese, sour cream, and cream cheese over full-fat ones, and mayonnaise made from canola oil instead of regular mayo. And in general, "if you're eating higher-fat foods, it's better [for your health] to eat the vegetable forms, versus animal fats," said Suhl.

So what does a balanced diet of nutritious foods for a healthy pregnancy actually mean? According to the American Dietetic Association, the March of Dimes, and womenshealth.gov, the U.S. federal government's source for women's health information, you should try to eat the following combination of foods each day:[7]

- **Protein and legumes:** two to three servings. A serving of protein is 2 to 3 ounces of cooked lean meat, poultry, or fish (about the size of a deck of cards), 2 tablespoons of peanut butter, ½ cup of tofu, 1 egg, or ½ cup of cooked dried beans. Keep an eye on the carb counts; legumes are typically higher in carbs than proteins, which have few to no carbs.

- **Dairy:** three to four servings (1,000–1,300 milligrams a day) each day. One serving of calcium is 1 cup (8 ounces) of milk, 1 cup of yogurt, 1½ ounces of natural cheese such as cheddar, or 2 ounces of processed cheese such as American. (Skim and low-fat varieties will help you avoid eating more fat than necessary.)

- **Fruits and vegetables:** seven servings combined. One fruit serving is 1 medium apple, 1 medium banana, 16 grapes, ½ cup of fresh, frozen, or canned fruit, ¾ cup of fruit juice, or ¼ cup of dried fruit. (A fruit serving typically has more carbs than a vegetable serving does.) One veggie serving equals 1 cup of raw leafy vegetables, ½ cup of other raw or cooked (nonstarchy) vegetables such as cucumbers, peppers, mushrooms, onions, garlic, beets, green beans, broccoli, celery, carrots, cauliflower, and tomatoes, or ¾ cup of vegetable juice. Keep an eye on the carb counts. Most vegetables are low in carbs, but don't forget to add them to your total carb count for a meal so that your insulin dose covers it. You need to take insulin even for a small healthy snack—one serving of baby carrots, about 14 pieces, is 8 grams of carb, for example. Starchier vegetables such as corn and potatoes are much higher in carbs (38 grams for two ears of corn and 51 grams for a medium baked potato with skin).

Organic Versus Nonorganic Foods

Foods made or grown without pesticides are considered organic; foods made or grown using conventional farming practices are considered nonorganic. Even when nonorganic foods are washed thoroughly, pesticide residues will likely remain on the surface. In addition, meat cuts from animals raised on nonorganic corn or grass are considered by some experts to be less healthy than those from animals raised organically, especially if the animals have also been injected with antibiotics to prevent diseases that are common on nonorganic feedlots. According to the U.S. Environmental Protection Agency, the many different kinds of pesticides cause a variety of health issues.[8] These include problems with the nervous system and the hormone or endocrine system, and skin or eye irritation. Other pesticides might be linked to cancer. Some experts say that organically raised beef and pork have higher nutritional value than nonorganic meat cuts. The idea is that you are not just what you eat but also whatever your food has eaten.

Should you buy organic foods? On one hand, pesticide residue might be harmful to a growing baby, and the potential effect is likely to be bigger in the baby's small body in utero than in your body. On the other hand, organic foods are often more expensive than their nonorganic counterparts, and they're not always as widely available. If you can't avoid eating nonorganic fruits and vegetables, it's a good idea to peel the skins. It's recommended that you buy organic versions of the following foods, often because it's tough to peel the skins or because the skins are thin: apples, bell peppers, celery, cherries, imported grapes, nectarines, peaches, pears, potatoes, raspberries, spinach, and strawberries.[9] It's not as important to buy organic forms of foods such as avocadoes and bananas, which are usually peeled anyway, if you need to make choices about what to buy. And while it's true that eating organic is always the healthier way to go, said Suhl, people have eaten nonorganic foods since the beginning of modern farming, and billions of babies whose mothers ate strictly conventional food have been born healthy.

- **Bread, cereal, rice, and pasta:** six to nine servings (one serving is 1 ounce or approximately 15 grams of carb). One serving equals 1 slice of bread, ½ cup of cooked cereal, rice, or pasta, or 1 cup of ready-to-eat cereal. Whole-grain versions typically have more fiber than white versions, and this helps keep postmeal blood sugars from spiking so high.

- **Iron:** foods high in iron include lean red meat, fish, poultry, dried fruits, whole-grain bread, and iron-enriched cereals. Talk to your doctor about whether you need an iron supplement in addition to your prenatal vitamin.

- **Salt:** for some of us, there's nothing better than a giant half sour deli pickle, pregnant or not. But use salt in moderation during pregnancy, as it can contribute to high blood pressure, fluid retention, bloating, and, in my case, the joy of cankles (ankles that are so swollen they look like calf extensions). Talk to your doctor about salt intake and heed what she says if you find yourself retaining water or if your blood pressure starts to climb.

What About Artificial Sweeteners?

According to Suhl, sucralose (sold under the brand name Splenda) is completely okay to use while you are pregnant (and when not pregnant). "It never gets into the blood," she said. "It stays in the digestive tract." Other products, including aspartame (brand name Equal) and saccharin (brand name Sweet'N Low), do get absorbed into the blood and are more likely to be absorbed by the fetus as well. "What we usually say is that one serving of food with aspartame per day is okay," while sucralose is fine anytime during pregnancy. While Suhl says that saccharin should be avoided during pregnancy, the American Dietetic Association says moderate saccharin intake is okay—use your own judgment if you want to eat saccharin.[10] If you want to avoid artificial sweeteners for whatever reason, consider using table sugar or honey in moderation. Count the extra carbs these sweeteners add to your meal, and take enough insulin to cover for the blood sugar rise.

- **Liquids:** at least eight 8-ounce glasses a day. Having enough fluids in your body helps flush your system and can help prevent constipation, hemorrhoids, urinary tract infections, dehydration, and swelling (the extra liquid moves salt out of your body). While water is great, you can also up your fluid intake by drinking milk, fruit juice (keep this in mind if you use juice to treat insulin reactions), decaf coffee and tea, soup, soda water, seltzer, and club soda.

What Not to Eat—Or At Least What to Think Twice About

Maybe you have an iron stomach and a steel constitution. Great. But your developing kid is a bit more fragile. The growing fetus can pick up illnesses from foods that have never given you any trouble before. It's because of these potential risks that most doctors in the United States tell pregnant women to avoid certain foods. Here's more of the lowdown from the March of Dimes and the Food and Drug Administration:[11]

- **Raw fish, such as sushi or sashimi, and shellfish such as clams or oysters.** Because these items aren't cooked, any bacterial content from raw sewage or other toxins won't be killed off. Such nastiness can give you severe stomach and digestive system woes. And yes, it's likely true that pregnant women in Japan and other places continue to eat sushi regularly and, presumably, have healthy children. Here in the United States, most docs prefer to be safe and recommend that you avoid sushi and sashimi altogether, rather than have you or your kid develop a problem after you eat a bad piece of raw fish. You can think the same thing about feta cheese in Greece, red wine in France, and other foods that are staples in other cultures but are considered off limits during pregnancy in the United States. It's up to you to make your own informed decisions about what health risks you are willing to take.

- **Fish high in mercury, particularly shark, swordfish, king mackerel, and tilefish.** Mercury, a metal that exists naturally in the environment, interacts with bacteria in water and can become toxic. Consuming too much mercury during pregnancy can cause problems with your unborn or young child's developing nervous system. While just about every fish has mercury in its body, the health benefits of eating certain low-mercury fish outweigh avoiding fish altogether because of the potential limited mercury exposure. Mercury content increases in fish as they move up the food chain (bigger fish eat smaller fish; mercury accumulates accordingly), which is why large fish such as shark, swordfish, king mackerel, and tilefish should be avoided while you are pregnant. The March of Dimes and the Food and Drug Administration recommend that pregnant women eat up to 12 ounces of fish such as shrimp, pollock, catfish, canned light tuna, salmon, herring, anchovies, sardines, and trout a week. Alternatively, you can eat up to 6 ounces of albacore (white) tuna per week. All these fish are good protein sources, and salmon, herring, anchovies, sardines, and trout in particular are rich in omega-3 fatty acids, which help nurture a child's brain growth.

- **Certain soft cheeses, such as Brie, blue-veined cheese, Camembert, Roquefort, feta, queso blanco and queso fresco; unpasteurized milk and dairy products; and ready-to-eat meats such as hot dogs, deli meats, refrigerated pates or meat spreads, and smoked seafood.** Listeriosis, a form of food poisoning, is the issue here. Bacteria in these foods can bring on flu-like symptoms that can quickly lead to meningitis or infections that result in a miscarriage, premature delivery, or stillbirth. Reheating the cheeses or deli meats to steaming-hot temperatures (a 10-second microwave zap is usually sufficient) will kill the bacteria and make the food safe to eat. If there's a particular soft cheese you like that's made in the United States, check whether it's made with pasteurized milk; if it is, it should be fine to eat. The hot dogs, some deli meats, and smoked foods are all made with nitrates, a preservative that isn't recommended during pregnancy. Talk to your doctor to see whether preservative-free alternatives (such as all-natural chicken sausages) are an acceptable substitute.

- **Raw or lightly cooked eggs (including soft-scrambled eggs, eggnog, Hollandaise sauce, Caesar salad dressing,**

and raw cookie dough or cake batters, including thosefound in some ice cream flavors) and rare or undercooked meat and poultry. These foods can cause listeriosis and other nasty foodborne illnesses such as salmonellosis, toxoplasmosis, or food poisoning from bacteria such as *Escherichia coli* or *Campylobacter* species. If a pregnant woman picks up one of these illnesses, the baby in utero can get even sicker from the infection. The results can range from diarrhea and fever to meningitis after the baby is born. Toxoplasmosis, an infection from parasites that come from infected cats, can cause vision and hearing loss, mental retardation, seizures, and other issues once the child is born. This is also why women should skip changing their cat's kitty litter box throughout pregnancy; get your partner to clean it out.

- **Raw vegetable sprouts (including alfalfa, clover, radish, and mung or bean sprouts) and unpasteurized fruit juice.** These can cause *Salmonella* and/or *E. coli* infections.

- **Liver.** Because of its high vitamin A content, liver is something you don't need to eat a lot of, particularly if you are taking a prenatal vitamin that is already giving you 100 percent of the vitamin A you need each day. Check with your doctor how much is healthy if you're a liver lover.

- **Caffeine.** Coffee, teas, chocolate, colas and other soft drinks, and some over-the-counter medications contain caffeine (and even decaf versions may have small amounts). The March of Dimes notes that up to 200 milligrams of caffeine a day (about the amount in 1½ cups of coffee) is generally considered safe. However, make sure your caffeine intake (a daily cup of coffee at breakfast, for example) doesn't replace other foods (such as a glass of skim milk at the same meal) that might provide more nutrients for you and your baby. Higher caffeine intake may be linked to miscarriage and stillbirth and to faster heart rates and other newborn health issues.

- **Alcohol.** Cutting alcohol out of your diet is the universal recommendation these days. Yes, yes, your French girlfriend continues to sip red wine *avec bébé*, but the research is pretty clear: alcohol can cause a laundry list of problems in the developing fetus, including mental retardation; learning, emotional, and behavioral problems; and defects in the face, heart, and other organs. Fetal alcohol syndrome, a mix of physical and mental birth defects, is the only form of mental retardation that is completely preventable by avoiding alcohol before and during pregnancy, according to the March of Dimes.

- **Herbal teas and herb supplements.** While some products are considered safe, others could be harmful. Check with your doctor about what is okay and what isn't.

- **Tobacco, marijuana, and other drugs.** I'm surely not the first to tell you that cigarettes, pot, cocaine, and any other illicit drugs are a totally bad idea during pregnancy—and also not so great when you're just trying to manage your diabetes even without a baby inside. The health risks of smoking, snorting, shooting, or eating such substances are numerous and preventable. If you use these drugs, stop. If you need help stopping, particularly before you get pregnant but especially after you are pregnant, talk to your doctor. Many resources can help you quit smoking or using drugs, and the benefits to you and your baby are immeasurable.

The Type 1/Type 2 Twist

Theoretically, you should be able to eat what you want, count the carbohydrates, and take a precise amount of insulin to control your blood sugar. In reality, diabetes can throw curve balls from out of nowhere, and pregnancy adds another element of potential surprise. What works for one woman might be completely unhelpful for another. Exercise, illness, and hormones in flux can make diabetes unpredictable and tough to manage.

"We are all different," said Elizabeth "Bjay" Woolley, 40, type 2, of Tuscon, Arizona. Her son is 8. "Track your carb counts per meal, and test, test, test to see what foods help you and which seem to be hindering you. Some people have parts of the day where blood sugars are hard to control, and others where they tend to run low. You can use this information to plan your menu or times you eat."

Woolley admitted that her diet changed "drastically" once she knew she was pregnant and got solid medical care. Diagnosed with type 2 in her early twenties, Woolley received no diabetes education about eating or diet other than what her clinic gave her in a pamphlet. "I figured the pills were all I needed," she said. "A typical meal for me then was fast food, meals from restaurants, or stuff from the store that came in boxes. I didn't pay attention at all to my meals; I just made what I felt like. So dinner could have been a Jumbo Jack [hamburger], fries, and a Diet Coke."

Several years later, Woolley sought advice about her pre-pregnancy diabetes concerns from the campus doctor at the university she was attending at the time. The doctor, not a diabetes specialist, merely told her "to have fun" when she asked whether there was anything she should do to prepare herself for a pregnancy with type 2 diabetes.

Two months later, she was pregnant and still thought she needed better diabetes care. She found a new team who helped her go on insulin and taught her about food and diabetes. "After I got pregnant, I was more conscientious," she said. "I paid attention to the sugar and carbs. I tried to have no more than one serving of carb per snack and two servings per meal. My foods were more fresh foods such as fruits and vegetables. A typical dinner was stir-fried veggies, chicken, and a roll. For breakfast, it was hard to find meals that wouldn't spike my sugars—I usually ate eggs and a corn tortilla. And for lunch, I tried to eat salads."

Talk to your doctor about any specifics if you're making significant changes in your diet as you prepare for pregnancy or while you are pregnant. A doc or a nutritionist might recommend that you limit your carb intake, for example, or suggest that you cut down on foods filled with animal fats. In short, pregnancy requires that you eat a well-balanced diet, adding only about 300 calories a day (in the second and third trimesters only) to give your baby the nutrients it needs.

Of course, it can be hard to eat well all the time, particularly if you didn't eat that way before you got pregnant. However, many women find that their motivation is strongest when they know they are carrying a baby.

"I tried to eat as if I were pregnant when I was trying to conceive, but I fell off that wagon each month," said Sharon, 34, type 1, of Pennsylvania. Her daughter is 4. "Once I really was pregnant though, I was able to stick to a much better routine," she said. "I had a gut instinct that I would be able to maintain the almost superhuman A1c levels when pregnant, and I was right about that."

Joy McCarren, 33, type 1, of Belle Center, Ohio, agreed. Now the mother of a 16-month-old, McCarren used an insulin pump and a CGM to help her fine-tune her blood sugar control and easily make adjustments in her insulin doses. Despite the ease of the technology, "it was very time consuming and at times felt like a full-time second job I was working. But knowing that keeping good control was the best thing for my baby, I had no qualms with doing so," she said.

Eating for two requires special considerations when blood sugar control is a factor. "I had already been eating very healthy before I got pregnant, but my diet changed because there were certain foods, like bananas and oatmeal, I could no longer eat because they made my blood sugar high regardless of how much insulin I took," said McCarren. Her attitude about meals that caused short blips of high blood sugars has changed, too. "Before I was pregnant, I wouldn't worry if I went out to eat or wanted pizza once in a while because I would guess how many carbs I was eating and take insulin accordingly," she said. "Once pregnant, I was very aware of everything I was eating and to the best of my ability ate things that I could know for certain what the carbs were."

Just Can't Get Enough: Dealing With Food Cravings (and Aversions)

Food foibles during pregnancy are well documented for some and don't bother others, but a few possible theories exist about why they occur. The flood of hormones coursing through your body may be one reason you suddenly want a particular food in the most insane way or an old favorite now sickens you. Another theory is that cravings are a sign of what your body needs more of, while aversions are a way to help you keep toxins out. Yet another theory suggests that you crave protein and certain vitamins at the beginning of your pregnancy because of which parts of the fetus are developing and that you want more fat toward the pregnancy's end because it's required by the developing brain. Whatever the reason, how do you handle cravings and aversions without crazy sugars to follow?

"I don't think it's unreasonable to give in, as long as your blood sugars are under control," said Emmy Suhl. If something is making

Carbs: Simple Versus Complex and the Glycemic Index

A carb isn't a carb isn't a carb when you're battling for blood sugar control. Different kinds of carbs cause blood sugars to do different things.

- Simple versus complex. A simple carb is a sugar, and a complex carb is a starch, said Emmy Suhl. It's the difference between a tablespoon of white cane sugar and a tablespoon of steel-cut oatmeal. The simple carb will typically cause your sugars to spike rapidly after eating, while the complex carb may cause a slower and less pronounced rise—often because of higher fiber content and less processing (although there are always exceptions for different people). It's more likely that injected or infused insulin will peak to better match a gradual blood sugar rise rather than a quicker one.

- Glycemic index, low versus high. The glycemic index (GI) is another way to measure how quickly a food can raise blood sugar levels.[12] Foods at the low end of the index, called low-glycemic foods, are less likely to raise blood sugar levels rapidly than those at the high end of the index, called high-glycemic foods. The amount of food you eat makes a difference as well. Low-GI foods include steel-cut oatmeal, hummus, edamame, beans, tofu, barley, sweet potatoes, whole-wheat pasta that's been cooked al dente, berries, apples, pears, grapefruits, whole-grain breads and crackers, foods with stone-ground wheat, and most vegetables. Often, foods high in fiber are considered low GI, as fiber helps slow the absorption of food into the blood and slow the rise of blood sugar after food is eaten. High-GI foods include those made with white flour, white rice, white potatoes, and white sugar (see a theme here?), doughnuts, corn chips, potato chips, waffles, puffed rice cereal, corn flakes, dates, and, oddly, watermelon.

you uncomfortable and a particular food that's considered healthy during pregnancy could make you feel better, then count the carbs, eat what you need to eat, and bolus or inject appropriately. If it's something less nutritious, eat within reason, bolus or inject the right amount of insulin, enjoy, and move on. "I was really able to eat anything I wanted with my insulin pump," said Allison Herschede, 29, type 1, of Hinesville, Georgia. Her kids are now 4 and 2. "I ate M&Ms every day and was able to keep my A1cs in the fives."

Sometimes a food craving or aversion is a sign of really low blood sugars. I once figured I had to be low when an orange-flavored Hostess cupcake looked awfully tempting (usually its overall fakeness seems gross), and a quick fingerstick proved me right. "I did have general food aversions from time to time, but they turned out to be an unusual symptom of severe low blood sugar," said Sharon. "The idea of any food was unappealing to me at all, and I didn't feel low otherwise. By the time it occurred to me or my family to test, I was 35 mg/dL."

Eating five or six smaller meals throughout the day, rather than three large meals and maybe a few snacks, can help keep things under control. "I ate small meals throughout the day and allowed myself good, healthy, low-carb snacks like sugar-free pudding," said Joy McCarren. "It helped to stave off any cravings."

Other times, though, the sky is the limit when it comes to what people desire and what they dislike:

- "I craved sushi with my first pregnancy, so I ate cooked sushi, California rolls, and tempura rolls," said Erin Argueta. "I had to adjust my insulin doses for sushi, because the rice wine vinegar does wreak havoc, but I maintained good blood sugars."

- "I craved hot, spicy foods like hot chicken wings, Mexican foods, hot peppers on pizza, and dairy foods like milk, cheese, and ice cream," said Amy Eddy, 33, type 1, from Utica, New York, and the mother of a 3-year-old son. "It didn't affect my sugars, though, because I tested over eight times a day anyway and was always bolusing."

- "I had minor cravings for foods that are substantial, like real cheddar cheese and steak," said Amy Mercer, 38, type 1, of Charleston, South Carolina, mom to two boys, ages 7 and 5, and halfway through her third pregnancy. "I also craved carb-heavy foods like breads, but I did my best to limit carb intake to meal time and snack on things like peanuts and rolled-up slices of turkey in between meals."

- "My eating habits didn't really change," said Jennifer Landers, 34, type 1, of Rochester Hills, Michigan. She is the mom to a toddler and halfway through her second pregnancy. "We were trying to conceive for almost two years, and I really worked with my docs that whole time to be in target range for my A1c and blood glucose readings, so once I got pregnant I just continued. With both pregnancies, the things I have craved the most are salad and veggies, so no effect on blood sugar!"

- "I definitely craved my old fast-food diet and junk food," said Michelle Kowalski. "I had shunned fast food nearly cold turkey because I was afraid to eat anything unhealthy. The first time I indulged in Tater Tots was like heaven."

- "I had cravings for waffles, pizza, bacon—most things that were bad," said Anna Tang Norton. "I kept cravings at bay; I satisfied them, but also made sure to eat healthy [the rest of the time]."

- "With my first pregnancy, I had cravings for pigs in the blankets [miniature hot dogs wrapped in pastry]," said Abby Nagel. "In the beginning, my sugars were okay, but I had to give them up in the second trimester due to the nitrates, and the fat just threw my sugars off completely."

- "I ate a lot of low-carb ice cream with strawberries, chocolate syrup, and peanuts—a couple times I ate that twice a day," said Traicy Lewis. "I ate Doritos, too, and peanut butter sandwiches on light wheat bread. I just bolused accordingly for everything."

Nausea and Your Numbers: Handling Morning Sickness

Some women never feel a hint of queasiness during their pregnancies, while others throw up so regularly they need to take medication to function. Whether you're somewhere in the middle of this spectrum or vomiting constantly, nausea needs to be monitored so that your insulin isn't peaking just after you've emptied your stomach. Some people said that morning sickness didn't affect their blood sugar levels; others recalled frequent lows and regular adjustments to insulin doses.

Morning sickness—incorrectly named, because it can last all day—refers to the nausea and/or vomiting experienced by about a third to a half of all pregnant women. According to the Mayo Clinic's website, nausea can be caused in part by the zooming amounts of estrogen in your body.[13] This can slow the absorption of food in your body way, way down. With pregnancy comes the potential to smell things more keenly, so certain odors might trigger nausea in a way they didn't before. Taking your prenatal vitamin or other meds at night, before bed, might help you keep things down and reduce your chances of feeling ill.

"I only had mild nausea," said Sharon. "The only way it affected my blood sugars was that I was munching on Saltines and similar crackers more often" to keep it at bay, and she had to account for the carbs consumed.

An insulin pump can be a great tool with morning sickness because you can easily reduce your basal rate to take less insulin if you feel you can't keep anything down. Talk to your doctor about when and for how long you should reduce your basal rate, although your own trial and error might help you figure out a morning sickness routine.

If you are having trouble keeping food down or have no appetite, it's a good idea to check yourself for ketones at least once a day to make sure you aren't spilling any. Ketones are a sign that your body is in starvation mode; talk to your doctor right away about what to do if this is the case for you.

"I never threw up, but I would get very nauseous," said Joy McCarren. "Being on the pump made a huge difference because if I didn't feel good and didn't want to eat, I could simply adjust my basal rates if needed."

Nausea can also vary from pregnancy to pregnancy. Jennifer Landers had none at all with her first but found morning sickness so much of a challenge with her second that her obstetrician prescribed Zofran, an antinausea medication. "Once I get going and can keep a little something in my stomach all day, I am fine," said Landers. "It definitely affected my blood sugars. I was running higher than my target numbers at the beginning when I was so sick, because I was afraid to take the insulin to cover the food before I knew it would stay down."

Sometimes, frequent lows (the result of vomiting or just in general) can bring on hypoglycemia unawareness, which means that the signs that typically tell you your blood sugar is dropping aren't as apparent as they once were.

"I was constantly throwing up and my blood sugars dropped" all the time, said Abby Nagel. "During my first trimester in my second pregnancy, my sugar dropped to 19 mg/dL and I passed out. I had been working at my desk reading a document and I could not make any sense of it. I kept reading it over and I could not understand why I couldn't comprehend it. I got more and more frustrated. I did not get that I was going really low and just remember ending up on the floor of my office. My officemates ran in when they heard me fall. They had to call an ambulance to take me to the hospital."

Knowing you're susceptible to more insulin reactions might be a good incentive to test your blood sugar even more frequently, to consider using a CGM, and to be more aware of the possibility that you're going low if anything feels off or different to you. It can also be a teachable moment.

"The first thing I did was give my entire office a lesson in how to suspend my insulin pump, and I showed them where my stash of apple juice boxes were located in my desk," said Nagel. "Next, I tested even more frequently to make sure I knew where I was all day long. I also made sure to constantly work with my endocrinologist in adjusting my carb counts and basal rates. Now that the CGM is available, I would recommend using it, especially during pregnancy."

Ever-Changing Insulin-to-Carb Ratios (and Basal Rates)

Throughout pregnancy, those swirling hormones cause your body to become more resistant to insulin at some times and more likely to use insulin efficiently at others. Things can certainly change from one woman to another, but, in general, you might notice that your insulin needs increase (or decrease) as soon as you realize you're pregnant, increase around weeks 20 to 26, increase even more in your third trimester, and then drop somewhat around week 37 or so. You might also find you need less insulin at the beginning of your second trimester.

Some of this is due to the placenta just doing its job. The placenta is an organ in the uterus that gives your kid all the nourishment it needs while in utero and filters out the baby's waste products. As the placenta grows, it makes the body more resistant to available insulin, which will require you to inject or infuse even more of the stuff. So if you used to take two units of insulin for a glass of milk, for example, maybe now you'll need four. Your insulin-to-carbohydrate ratio might start increasing (along with basal rates if you're on an insulin pump) in your second trimester, and by the third trimester you might be taking in double or triple the insulin you did before (or even higher multiples).

This is totally normal. Don't be alarmed.

When my insulin doses started climbing, after recording some of the lowest blood sugar averages on my glucose meter I'd ever seen, I simply took whatever amount of insulin I needed to cover for the meal and moved on. One nondiabetic woman asked me whether I should eat less so that I wouldn't have to take as much insulin. I just told her that her body was doing the same thing as mine—she just didn't know it because her pancreas was doing all the work.

Knowing that your insulin requirements are going to increase can help you avoid getting freaked out or worse about needing so much insulin to keep your sugars under control.

"My increases started about four months into my pregnancy and tapered off toward the end, around 36 weeks," said Anna Tang Norton. "My ratio was high and I would change my basal rates in the doctor's office after checking my blood sugar and food logs. I never was irritated with all the changes—I was really mentally prepared for the worst during my pregnancy."

With all the changing details, even subsequent pregnancies can vex the veterans. "I remember the resistance being very frustrating," said Amy Mercer, now pregnant for the third time. "I have not quite reached the point where I need to start increasing with this pregnancy, but I know I will soon! [With my first two,] by the time I'd reached the end of my pregnancies, I was giving nearly three times the amount of insulin as I was at the beginning. I often felt like I couldn't eat anything, that any food I put in my mouth would spike my blood sugars, and, of course, I worried about what high sugars would do to the baby." Mercer's A1cs were in the 4 to 5 percent range for her previous pregnancies, so the increasing insulin amounts kept her average sugars well managed. Still, she admitted, "it took a lot of work."

Notes for a Nutritionist Appointment

You and your doctor may find it helpful for you to see a nutritionist with a diabetes background. Whether you need fine-tuning or a complete overhaul or just have some questions about eating, diabetes, and pregnancy, make sure that the expert you meet with has a solid understanding of the differences between type 1, type 2, and gestational diabetes. People with gestational diabetes don't always go on insulin and therefore may be told to eat a strict diet with limited carbs. Being on insulin gives you more flexibility about how many carbs you can eat and how you can cover their blood sugar effects with an insulin-to-carb ratio. At the same time, even though eating many carbs and giving yourself a lot of insulin to cover for them will likely keep your blood sugars in line, you'll probably gain weight (beyond simple baby or pregnancy pounds) with the extra calories.

"I learned about better whole wheats, smart butters, organic peanut butters, and other alternatives to regular foods that wouldn't send my blood sugar into a tailspin," said Michelle Kowalski. Her CDE taught her that whole-wheat or whole-grain breads can help smooth out blood sugars because their higher fiber content helps slow the transition from carbs to blood glucose. Foods such as peanut butter are likely to be healthier when they are made only from ground peanuts and a bit of oil rather than a commercial brand that has added sugars and hydrogenated fats, which require extra insulin and can raise your cholesterol levels.

Then again, if you've lived a long time with diabetes, it can be tempting to think that you have probably heard everything there is to know about eating and that a nutritionist visit would be a little been there, done that. Believe me, I've felt that way. But others have found it helpful.

"I was used to eating on the run and not very healthily," said Tracy Scoggins, 28, type 1, of Macomb, Illinois. She is halfway through her pregnancy with her third child, and her daughters are 5 and 3. "The nutritionist got me on a meal plan that would be both healthy for me and healthy for the baby. The advice they gave was helpful because they explained *why* I needed to eat the different kinds of food suggested and not just skip out on certain items. I can see a huge difference when I follow the meal plan that they set up and when I slack off."

Because eating while pregnant is probably different from how you usually eat, it's likely you'll learn something new. Despite her three pregnancies and 17 years of living with type 1 diabetes, Scoggins said her nutritionist appointments have been helpful. "I would recommend seeing a nutritionist because your body is going through many changes. What you were eating before conception won't be the same as what you are eating during your pregnancy. Information changes from year to year, so even if you saw a nutritionist for one pregnancy, the information and knowledge they have years down the road might change."

Whether or not your obstetrician can give you the latest information, "you'll want to know what the latest recommendations are for food contaminations," added Joslin Center nutritionist Emmy Suhl. "Science is always changing, with new insulins, new blood glucose monitors, and new insulin delivery devices. We now know more about how food affects blood glucose levels. If you want to optimize your blood sugar control, it's a good idea to see a nutritionist."

From the Mouths of Babes: The People Speak About How and What They Eat

You can listen to all the advice a doctor or nutritionist or CDE can offer, but sometimes there's nothing more helpful or satisfying than hearing what a woman did who has walked in the shoes you're in right now (swollen feet, cankles, and all).

"Try and look at the big picture instead of the hour-by-hour or meal-by-meal results," said Amy Mercer. "It's important to remember not to beat yourself up when you get a high blood sugar after a meal. I think food is such a complex issue for women with diabetes, and pregnancy just adds another layer." Managing diabetes involves an ongoing set of decisions and thoughts about what you ate last, what you'll eat next, how much insulin (if any) is working in your system, whether you plan to exercise, and what emotions or hormones are doing at any given time—so much so that it can be incredibly frustrating to deal with an out-of-range number, particularly right after a meal, when the numbers are more likely to go high.

For women with diabetes, "food and pregnancy is a complex roller coaster," said Jennifer Landers. "Foods that you thought you had figured out can have a different effect when pregnant. So test a lot more than you think you need to, and make corrections often." And to counteract more frequent low blood sugars, always have a ready food or glucose supply. "I keep a couple of granola bars stashed everywhere—in my purse, my desk, my car, my nightstand, and so on, along with glucose tabs or juice. Those lows can really sneak up on you fast."

It can be alarming to see a high number at any time, but particularly an hour after a meal, and my instinct was always to correct that high immediately. However, correcting before your meal insulin has had a chance to work—which typically takes a few hours, depending on the reaction time of your particular insulin—can lead to going low right away. "This reactive approach leads to blood glucoses that bounce from high to low," said Florence Brown, MD, codirector of the Diabetes and Pregnancy program at Joslin-Beth Israel Deaconess Medical Center and an instructor at Harvard Medical School, both in Boston, Massachusetts. "It is important to avoid treating high blood glucose if there is still insulin on board, as blood glucoses may crash when boluses are stacked. Adjustments to the insulin-to-carb ratios and basal rates should be made after clear patterns have been established. Ideally, if the basals and insulin-to-carb ratios are accurate and carb counting is accurate, one would not need to correct. On the other hand, sickness or pump catheter occlusion should be addressed immediately."

For me and many others, the reality is that lows happen often, particularly when you are trying so hard to stay within the recommended blood sugar ranges for pregnancy. It is important always to have some kind of fast-acting carbohydrate on hand to treat an insulin reaction at any time.

If you're out in public and find yourself going low without any source of glucose on you, consider condiments. If the line to buy a bottle of juice at a coffee shop or fast-food restaurant is long and winding, try going straight to the area where you can gets napkins and plastic forks. Sugar packets are usually there for the taking, and they're a quick and free way to get something into you fast. (One sugar packet is about 6 grams of carb.) If you feel guilty about taking sugar, go ahead and stand in the line at the register (after treating your low and knowing that your blood sugars are coming back up). You can always buy a bottle of water to ease your conscience, and it's better than waiting in an endless line to buy juice when you're sweating, feeling weak, and cursing the people ahead of you for counting out exact change from their penny collections.

No matter what you're eating, it's helpful to keep detailed and accurate records of what you eat, the carb counts, your insulin doses (basals and boluses on pumps), and your blood sugar numbers. It's tedious, and in this day of CGMs, wireless pump–meter relationships, and other downloadable data, you might be able to transfer some of the information to your computer and fax or e-mail it directly to your endocrinologist. But some docs are still old school and want to see paperwork, so keeping good records can help you achieve great control.

"Write everything down," said Abby Nagel. "If you have a flukey reading, you will know what you did [to get it]. It is hard to keep it all on track if you don't. I found it extremely helpful to fax my readings and food intake to my endo on almost a daily basis, to keep me on track."

This can work if you really want to eat something that's not jam-packed with vitamins and nutrients every once in a while, too. While pregnant, I worked full time in an office that a coworker stocked with miniature chocolates and other candies. I experimented with the low-er-fat items (I ate Peppermint Patties more often than, say, Reese's Peanut Butter Cups) and was able to figure out the carb counts, exact insulin ratios, and results of eating a small handful of these treats most days the candy was available (that is to say, nearly every day I worked). My blood sugars behaved well.

Keeping detailed records can help you figure foods out, too. "I kept a food journal during my pregnancy that helped me in several ways," said Joy McCarren. "It was an invaluable tool to have for trying new foods or even testing how foods I ate pre-pregnancy affected me during pregnancy. I would write down what I was eating, the carb totals, the calories if I knew them, my blood sugars, and any other info or note of interest. I know I will find it useful again when I am pregnant next time. Holidays were the hardest, but having the pump helped me to get through them with no major blood sugar issues."

Of course, balancing a healthy diet with the occasional small treat should be fine for your baby, provided you're taking your prenatal vitamins, testing your sugars, monitoring your insulin, and eating well. "I think one of the best things to keep in mind is that it's okay to indulge in treats every now and then," said Michelle Kowalski. "If you continue to deny yourself something, you may wind up obsessing over it or bingeing on it later. I think we have to remember not to beat ourselves up about every out-of-range blood sugar, because there will be out-of-range blood sugars. As long as your blood sugar isn't consistently out of range and you're not consistently eating poorly then it's okay."

Some people alter their eating habits not only for blood sugar control but also to feel better. "My eating habits didn't change right when I knew I was pregnant, because I thought I'd be fine eating the way I was," said Traicy Lewis. "I made the decision to eat six times a day at four months into my pregnancy. Around that time, I kept having lows and just was overly tired. This happens, but I thought I could do something about not feeling so drained." Her sister, who already had two children, suggested Lewis eat more frequently. It did the trick. "When I did that I felt so much better, even though I was *never* hungry. I ate my regular meals but also ate a 15 to 20 gram carb snack in between. I also had a snack before going to bed. I just bolused accordingly."

Where you eat can make a difference in how your sugars behave, too. "Try to eat mostly at home," said Heidi Wickstrom, 37, type 1, of Orange County, California. Her daughter is 2. "Try to skip a lot of eating out, especially fast foods." If you prepare food at home, you know exactly what's in it. Restaurant meals may have hidden oils, sugars, or thickeners in sauces that might affect your postmeal blood sugar readings. Portions are also notoriously large when you eat out; planning to eat only part of your entrée, or asking to take half the meal home, can help you keep meal serving sizes in check.

Ultimately, what you eat will sustain your child and you for the next nine-plus months (and longer if you plan to breast-feed, but let's take things one day at a time). It's a big responsibility, but you can handle it. "Being aware that what I put in my mouth ultimately nourished my child helped remind me to go for the healthy choices as opposed to the empty calories and processed carbs," said Joy McCarren. "There will be some days that you are much better controlled than others. On the days where it is harder to eat well, remember that the occasional high is not bad for the baby—it is the sustained highs you need to worry about. Relax and remember that even if you eat in the most healthy way possible, you will still have times where your blood sugars are out of range. That is unavoidable during pregnancy. Finding a good peer group online or a local support group can be invaluable as well in helping to get new food ideas and having others to talk to who are either in the same situation or have been there."

4

Tests and Bloods and Rockin' Goals: Pregnancy Assessments and Prenatal Exams

No doubt about it—having type 1 or type 2 diabetes puts you into the high-risk pregnancy category these days, even if you have the best control your doctors have ever seen. But don't get annoyed about a couple of words strung together. Instead, settle in and revel in the extra attention. You'll likely undergo a lot of tests to make sure things are progressing well. Here's the scoop on what they are, what they indicate, and whether you can opt out of some of them. And for times when things aren't typical, here's advice on carrying more than one baby, dealing with bed rest, finding a midwife who is willing to work with a woman with pre-existing diabetes, and more.

Testing, Testing

The number of doctor's appointments you'll be scheduled for will likely increase once you're officially pregnant. A lot of this is for monitoring—of your blood sugars, your A1cs, your developing fetus, and your own health. It's also to powwow with your doctors about any questions or issues you have and to see whether anything warrants a change in your routine, your insulin doses, your food intake, and so on. Your endocrinologist will order blood tests, and you'll likely pee in a cup and do a fingerstick to check your home meter's accuracy every time you visit the endo and the obstetrician. Your obstetrician will also usually ask for blood and urine and do ultrasounds, which are images taken of the developing baby—either vaginally in the earliest weeks of pregnancy or, later, using a wand that glides over your growing abdomen. Depending on what is typical for all patients in your doctor's office and what is offered specifically because of your diabetes (and what you choose to undergo or to decline), other exams can include the diagnostic tests to determine the risk of your baby having Down syndrome and trisomy 18, tests such as chorionic villus sampling (CVS) and amniocentesis to confirm whether there are chromosomal defects, a fetal echocardiogram to see potential heart problems, blood tests such as the quad screen, which shows the potential for neural tube defects, and a level 2 ultrasound to examine growing body parts.

Dealing With More Doctor's Appointments

By the time I had my son, I thought my hospital should have renamed itself the Cheryl Alkon Medical Center because I was there so often. (I certainly paid enough in insurance co-payments and parking fees to fund a plaque above a cushy area in the lobby.) You will likely visit your doctors' offices and the medical centers they practice out of many times. It's a good idea to be friendly, or at least halfway pleasant, to the office staff, the parking people, and anyone else you interact with regularly during these trips. You've got enough to think about with your own week-by-week issues with pregnancy, so why make a name for yourself as the patient who got cranky in the parking garage or the one who's snippy to the office staff? You're going to see them again and again.

Some people revel in the additional time and attention they get with the extra visits to the endocrinologist and obstetrician. Many appreciate the additional information provided during these meetings.

"I was totally okay with the extra appointments because they were more reassurance for me that everything was okay," said Amy Eddy. "I got to have more sonograms and nonstress tests than the average expectant mother, which kept me at ease." For some, the extra hassle and expense of long-distance travel are worth it for the info gleaned at the appointments. "I liked the extra attention and felt if there were any problem, diabetes related or not, I would know," said Sasha Boak Kelly, 38, type 1, of Hudson, New York. Her daughters are 3½ and 1. "I drove four hours roundtrip once a month or so for most of my pregnancies alone, including the eighth month. That got to be a drag, but I did not feel resentful, just purposeful—to have and do so much to get as good result as possible."

But like pregnancy itself, nine-plus months of doctor's appointments can get tedious. "At first it was sort of novel," said Alycia Green, 33, type 2, of Joliet, Illinois. Her son is 6 months old. "I definitely got more attention and questions from people about why I had all the appointments. I also loved having more frequent ultrasounds and images to bring home—that was the best part. Halfway through the pregnancy, the novelty began wearing thin, and by the end of the pregnancy, I didn't want to go to another doctor's office, period. I felt like that was all I was doing—hopping from one doctor to the next. Even with insurance, the co-pays really start to add up, and trying to take time off of work was a *big* pain."

Ah, yes. Trying to schedule appointments around your work hours can be a challenge if you don't work for yourself or if you have a rigid timetable at your job. Depending on your schedule, lining up the first or the last appointment of the day—even for several visits in advance if you can swing it—can help. Consider using your sick, personal, or vacation days if your boss or schedule isn't flexible enough to work around multiple medical visits (even though sitting in a doctor's office waiting to be seen is a far cry from lying on a sunny beach). If necessary, your endocrinologist, obstetrician, or any other doc you see can write a letter of medical necessity to your boss or employer to explain your need for time off for appointments. And if it is necessary to fight an employer's disapproval (or worse) of the time you need to take off during pregnancy, the U.S. Family and Medical Leave Act states that if you work for a company with 50 or more employees, any elementary or secondary school, or any public entity, you are allowed up to 12 weeks of unpaid time off for prenatal medical care (or pregnancy or childcare) without fear of losing your job or other repercussions.[1] (Not that you want to be dealing with a lawsuit or the potential for one while you're managing your pregnancy, but the law exists in case you need it.)

"I wasn't resentful, but I won't deny that it was stressful" to juggle all the visits, said Bethany Rose, 30, type 1, of Winnipeg, Manitoba, in Canada. Her daughter is 2 months old. "I missed a *lot* of work for appointments, but I was lucky that my boss was very understanding and that most of my appointments were within a few blocks' radius of my office building." Rose left her full-time job a few weeks before giving birth. However, "even though I was off work, it felt like these appointments were almost a full-time job," she said. "I seemed to have one or two every day." With the scheduling came reassurance, though.

"I felt very supported by a great medical team, from my obstetrician, to my endocrinologist, to my ophthalmologist, and so on," she said. "I definitely didn't feel like I did this alone."

Clearly, these visits eat up a lot of time. It's particularly tough when appointments run long and the wait times grow.

"I hated going to the doc more because I'd be there *forever*," said Kathryn, 42, type 1, of Georgia. Her twin daughters are 4. "But that was an issue with my particular endo practice. I don't understand why faxing in my blood glucose numbers and having a phone consult wouldn't work just as well. It would have saved me the time sitting in the waiting room. As soon as my pregnancy was over, I switched offices."

Blood and Urine Tests, Diabetes-Style

Holding out your arm to offer up a juicy vein and peeing into a plastic cup are standard routines at the typical endocrinologist appointment. They continue when you're seeing docs on the pregnancy circuit. The A1c tests also continue, but because the readings show the past two to three months of blood sugar control, you may not have a test on each visit if you're being seen every month or more frequently.

And while all pregnant women are handing over cups of urine to their doctors, some of us are collecting it in a jug at home for a 24-hour version or peeing on little plastic strips every morning. All these urine tests are checking to see whether your kidneys are functioning properly or whether your body is producing ketones in response to inadequate caloric intake or high blood sugars. At the beginning of pregnancy, a microalbumin test checks to see whether your kidneys are spilling tiny amounts of a protein called albumin, which is a sign of early kidney damage. Large amounts of albumin in the urine may indicate more advanced kidney disease. In addition, creatinine is a waste product filtered by your kidneys that accumulates in the blood if your kidneys aren't working right. When blood glucose numbers are very high because of inadequate insulin, such as after a missed insulin dose or pump catheter blockage, you will be asked to check for ketones, which are byproducts the body makes when it uses fat for energy instead of carbohydrates. High ketones can lead to diabetic ketoacidosis, which can be life-threatening. Diabetic ketoacidosis can happen at lower blood sugar levels if you are pregnant than if you are not pregnant.

As your pregnancy progresses, your doctor may ask you to do daily ketone checks at home using strips that you dip into your urine when you first get up to pee in the morning, or earlier in your pregnancy if you have severe morning sickness and can't keep anything down. And of course, glucose spilled into the urine means your blood sugars are high, but the blood sugar readings you get from actual blood using a portable monitor are far more accurate than those from urine, which can be hours old and not reflect the fact that your current blood sugar reading is within range.

As always, it is the average, long-term management of your blood sugar levels, not a high reading here and there, that is most important for the ongoing good health of your baby and you.

"Sometimes it came back that there was a lot of sugar in my urine, which some made a big deal about, but I didn't panic about it because I knew my blood glucose numbers were, for the most part, in very good control," said Traicy Lewis. "As far as I knew, all pregnant women had ongoing urine tests," said Bronwyn Florens, 30, type 1, of Johannesburg, South Africa. Her daughter is 22 months old. "They seemed less concerned when I had a bit of sugar in my urine than they had seemed when my pregnant sister who is not diabetic had the same thing." (All pregnant women have a lower renal threshold, which is why many of them spill glucose into their urine.)

Pre-Existing Kidney Complications

If you already had kidney issues before getting pregnant, you may see a nephrologist to monitor your kidneys throughout the pregnancy. You may need to forgo some medications that aren't recommended during pregnancy and while breast-feeding. You should follow up with your doctor immediately after having your baby to talk about when you can resume the medications so that your kidneys aren't further compromised.

Women who have had diabetes for a while—say, 20 years or longer—and who also have hypertension or kidney disease are more likely to be monitored for babies that are underweight than for overweight babies. The blood vessels around their placenta may have problems that can restrict the baby's growth. Regular ultrasounds around weeks 24 to 26 are typical to observe whether the baby is thriving and developing on schedule.

With all the extra blood sugar testing (and possibly the use of a CGM), it's likely that your average blood sugar readings will fall into a nice tight range—or at least a lower one than you're used to—during pregnancy.

"My A1c went down dramatically, because for the first time in my life, I was actually taking care of my diabetes and doing everything I was supposed to—everything my doctors have asked me to do for years," said Star Lewis, 26, type 1, of Allen, Oklahoma. Her sons are 6 and 7. "Getting pregnant saved my life."

Carrying a baby is a giant motivator to achieve and maintain what seem like impossible blood sugar goals. "The knowledge that someone was really counting on me to be in good control helped me test so much more often, and correct much sooner," said Sharon. "When not pregnant, I average a 7.5 A1c or so, but while pregnant, I was 5.4 and 5.6 the entire time."

It can be fantastic to watch your A1cs come down to levels you never thought possible before. "When I got my A1c down to 5.1 during pregnancy, I was elated," said Alycia Green. "I felt great, and I felt like I was doing everything that I was supposed to. I was proud of myself and felt this was greatly beneficial to my child."

Your doctor will also take blood at your first prenatal appointment, as is done for all pregnant women, with or without diabetes.[2] This blood is used for a bunch of tests:

- A complete blood count to measure the hemoglobin and various cell counts, which will indicate whether you have infections and how your iron measures up.

- Tests of your blood type and Rh factor. This will tell you whether your blood is Rh-positive or Rh-negative. If it's negative and your baby's blood is Rh-positive, your body may consider the developing baby a foreigner and the baby can develop anemia. This combination also can lead to fetal brain damage or death. This can be prevented with a shot of a product called Rh immunoglobulin, which is typically given at 28 weeks or following an amniocentesis.

- An antibody screen, which will indicate whether you have any antibodies that have developed from an earlier pregnancy or a blood transfusion.

- Tests to see whether you are immune to rubella (German measles) or have syphilis, hepatitis B, or HIV.

- Kidney function and liver function tests to ensure the levels are normal at the beginning of your pregnancy in case you develop high blood pressure later in the pregnancy.

- Tests to ensure your thyroid hormone readings are in the normal range.

- A test of creatinine level to evaluate kidney function.

Blood work is common throughout the pregnancy, and it's not just for A1c tests. Around weeks 34 through 36, you're typically screened for group B strep, a bacteria found in the vagina that can require the use of antibiotics during labor so that the strep doesn't infect the baby. "Group B strep bacteria is found more often in patients with diabetes, but it is a highly preventable infection for the baby when monitored and treated," said Tamara Takoudes, MD, codirector of the Diabetes and Pregnancy program at Joslin-Beth Israel Deaconess Medical Center and a clinical instructor at Harvard Medical School.

Understanding Ultrasounds

Depending on the protocol at your doctor's office and the specifics of your pregnancy, you may have anywhere from a couple of ultrasounds, to several, to so many that you lose count before you actually give birth. Ultrasounds are an easy way to see how your baby is thriving inside you. Just before I got pregnant, one nondiabetic woman told me she wanted to minimize the number of ultrasounds she had for her second pregnancy because of the possibility they could "heat the womb." Ultrasounds have been used for a few decades, and to date they have not been linked to any risks to either mother or baby, so that theory doesn't seem to hold water. "Ultrasound has no known risk," said Dr. Ian Grable. "They have been used since the 1960s and they seem to have no negative effects on babies during pregnancy." For a high-risk pregnancy, an ultrasound by a trained sonographer or radiologist can provide much information about whether your child is progressing properly and when medical care might be necessary, either in utero or immediately after giving birth. "Ultrasound is a powerful screening tool used in all pregnancies, but when a patient has diabetes, it can detect physical birth defects in the fetus and gauge the well-being of the fetus in later pregnancy," said Dr. Tamara Takoudes.

Women with diabetes typically get more ultrasounds than women without diabetes. Some are particularly happy about the practice. "I got to actually watch my babies grow right in front of me," said Star Lewis. "Most women get ultrasounds done only a couple times. I felt so lucky and so much closer to my baby with each pregnancy" because of the extra ultrasounds.

However, most doctors refrain from giving ultrasounds to anyone just for the heck of it, in part to minimize any potential risk to the baby in utero, but also because there may be no medical reason to do so. Without a medical reason, insurance companies will not cover the cost of the test. Double check with your doc if you want to get (and pay for) an ultrasound for fun outside the medical realm, such as in a shopping mall or at a celebrity's home. (In 2005, actor Tom Cruise reportedly bought an ultrasound machine for his then-girlfriend, actress Katie Holmes, to check on their daughter, Suri, in utero while at their residence.) "This is absolutely not recommended because Tom Cruise is not certified to use ultrasound safely," said Dr. Tamara Takoudes. "Ultrasound for entertainment is not medically necessary and can cause harm when done improperly or too often."

There are other concerns about getting one of these photos. "In general, [these shopping mall businesses] make you sign a waiver that says if they find an abnormality, they won't tell you," said Dr. Ian Grable. "I have significant problems with places that might see a problem and won't tell you."

The level 2 ultrasound is a detailed look at all your baby's organs and parts and measures the baby's age in utero. This test is typically done between weeks 17 and 22, and it's exciting because you (or the technician doing the scan) can see what's what and can learn such things as whether your baby's legs are longer or shorter than average. It is also the appointment when, if the baby isn't shy, you can learn whether you're having a boy or a girl.

"I had nine ultrasounds during my pregnancy," said Bronwyn Florens. "One was with a specialist neonatologist at the 20-week scan for a better check for abnormalities. This was something that was not required in the average pregnancy. Nothing was ever out of the ordinary. I was aware that towards the end they checked the baby's size

Managing Multiples

Sometimes ultrasounds can give you the news that you're carrying more than one fetus. This may be a surprise, or it may be a possibility you were already aware of if you underwent fertility treatment.

Twin (or higher) pregnancies with pre-existing diabetes can be more of a challenge because of the extra stress on your body. Talk to your doctor about how much more you should eat and how your insulin needs will reflect that. You'll likely need more monitoring than for a singleton pregnancy. "We do ultrasounds, the level 2 ultrasound and regular ultrasounds for growth, and nonstress tests in the third trimester," said Dr. Ian Grable. "The biggest issue is preterm labor, so there's a lot of monitoring the cervix. It adds a level of complexity to the pregnancy. With twins and two placentas, it adds more insulin resistance, so there's more insulin requirements along with vigilant blood sugar monitoring."

Kathryn's twin girls were diagnosed in utero with a rare condition called twin-to-twin transfusion syndrome. (The babies shared one placenta; the condition can lead to cord blood issues and congestive heart failure. It was *not* related to her diabetes.) She spent much of her pregnancy on bed rest and delivered at 32 weeks. The girls are now 4 and healthy.

"My diabetes, because I had so many other problems going on, was something I could control, and it made me happy I could control it," she said. "I checked my blood sugar 12 times a day. My insurance company was being a poop ass about my strips, so my father, who has type 2 and didn't test as often as I did, called and got a prescription for more test strips, which I used."

Her best advice for a multiple mom-to-be is to be proactive and learn all you can. "Educate yourself about twin pregnancy," she said. "Don't get scared. Yes, it's hard—I'm not going to blow smoke up anyone's behind. But it's doable and it's doable without full-time help." More tidbits from Kathryn:

- It's not uncommon to lose one twin in a twin pregnancy.
- "If you don't know how to count carbs, learn. If you're not on an insulin pump, you're crazy," she said. You may be able to make an argument to your insurance company that it is medically necessary if your insurance

company denies your first request. (The same could be said for getting coverage for a CGM during pregnancy.) However, some doctors note that certain women are not candidates for an insulin pump because they don't have the skills or motivation to use the pump effectively. Other pregnant women do very well with multiple daily injections, particularly those with type 2, who have relatively more stable blood sugars than type 1 women. Insurance companies might not cover insulin pumps for type 2 women despite appeals. Talk to your doc about what is best for you.

- Boiled eggs are your best friend. "I ate a lot of protein and veggies, and less fruit and almost no pasta. I ate full-fat ice cream before bed. I was cheesed out and peanut butter didn't taste right. Staying hydrated was hard—I drank Crystal Light and decaf iced tea with lots of lemon. Don't freak out about Splenda." (However, you may find that eating high-fat foods at bedtime makes overnight blood sugars harder to control.)

- Join a twin club while you're pregnant, even if the one closest to you is across the state. These clubs provide a wealth of information and give you a place to vent about a dumb remark you heard someone make about twins.

- If you need to go back to work, start visiting childcare programs as soon as you find out you are pregnant. Even if you want a nanny, look into different programs. In-home daycares are easier to get for twins than pre-school spaces.

- "The hardest thing about parenting with twins is Mommy brain—remembering to test my blood sugar. My kids now ask me to test their blood sugar because they want to do what Mom is doing. It's probably a good idea to teach them to remind me to test my own sugar once they get older."

more than they might have in a normal pregnancy, and they were also checking more for calcification of the placenta."

Early ultrasounds also might give you news you aren't expecting—that there is a problem. While the number of potential problems is a topic for another book, getting as much information as you can from your doctor and through your own informed, scientific research (and not something you find on some dodgy website without solid sources) will help you make an educated decision about how to fix or work with the issue. And sometimes, things resolve on their own.

"I had seven ultrasounds," said Joy McCarren. "My doctors discovered a slight placental separation and they monitored that closely, but it never changed. I'd had bleeding at 12 weeks and was put on bed rest. They believe that is when the separation occurred, but it never got any worse."

Multiple Marker Tests

Multiple marker tests, which are often optional, determine your child's risk for developing certain birth defects. Depending on your age and other factors, the risk of a false positive can be higher than your actual risk. Talk with your doctor about the relative benefits of doing these or skipping them. Some people want as much additional information about their pregnancies as they can get; others don't want the stress of potential false-positive results. And some people feel that they will love and care for a baby regardless of whatever genetic or other issues the child might have, so there's no point in screening for anything beforehand.

With screening tests, "I had it all," said Sasha Boak Kelly. "My A1cs were not perfect before becoming pregnant, and the tests were recommended" because all the major organs form during the first eight weeks of pregnancy. When both her first and second pregnancies revealed no abnormal test results, she said, "I was relieved."

People's opinions can change as the pregnancy progresses. "I did one round of tests for birth defects," said Lindsay Gopin. "After this came back normal, I did not want to proceed with further testing. I thought it was too overwhelming, and I had heard a lot of stories of false-positive results."

Still others change their minds in favor of the tests after more discussion. "I wasn't going to get the tests done at first, and my OB/GYN was fine with that," said Alycia Green. "But another doctor recommended I get one done, and he scared me into it, describing all the possible birth defects. Initially, I do not believe I would have terminated the pregnancy unless there was something very drastic, so I didn't think it was necessary. But I am glad that I did [the test]. I would have felt awful if there was a problem that could have been dealt with throughout the pregnancy." Testing can give you information about a potential complication ahead of time so that you can better prepare for the delivery and ensure that all the medical personnel required for your baby's condition are available on site when the infant is born.

The first-trimester combined screen or early risk assessment is done around weeks 9 through 13. It typically includes an ultrasound to measure the thickness of the back of your baby's neck. This is the nuchal translucency test, and the result can indicate the risk that your child might have chromosomal abnormalities such as Down syndrome, congenital heart defects, or other genetic issues. The blood work done with this screen tests for two hormones called PappA and human chorionic gonadotropin (hCG) and will also indicate the risk for Down syndrome and another common chromosomal disorder, trisomy 18.

Quad screens, done around weeks 15 through 20, measure the levels in the mother's blood of four things that are secreted by the fetus: alpha-fetoprotein (AFP), hCG, estriol, and inhibin-A. A quad screen can test for Down syndrome or trisomy 18 if you missed the early test. (A triple screen measures only three factors.) The AFP part of this blood test can indicate the level of risk that your baby has a neural tube defect or a chromosomal problem. Women with diabetes are more at risk for having babies with neural tube defects (though the risks go down the closer your A1cs are to normal ranges). The AFP test has a different range of normal results for women with diabetes, so make sure it is clearly marked on the test that you have it; otherwise, false positives are common.

"We chose, with the help and support of our perinatologist, to only have the AFP test done," said Sharon. "We knew there wasn't anything that a birth defect would change in our mind, but the peri helped us realize that if a defect existed in the spinal cord and we knew about it, we'd be able to discuss having a surgeon at the delivery. We also discussed a new in vitro surgery that was available in our area. My biggest fear was actually of false positives. I didn't expect any real issues, but I was worried I'd get a false positive and then have to go through a chorionic villus sampling [CVS] or amnio to confirm or disprove the results."

Depending on your age and the results of these screens, your doctor might suggest more invasive prenatal testing, such as CVS or amniocentesis.

Invasive Prenatal Tests: What's Up in There

CVS is recommended in a small number of patients—typically, if you're 38 or older or have certain genetic conditions that increase the risks associated with having a baby. CVS can reveal whether your baby has Down syndrome, Tay-Sachs, sickle-cell anemia, and most types of cystic fibrosis. This test usually happens around weeks 10.5 to 13, and it is considered highly accurate. Your doctor will take a small sample of tissue from the placenta and test it for genetic problems. The tissue can be obtained vaginally or using a needle inserted through the abdomen; both procedures use ultrasound to identify exactly where the doctor will obtain the tissue from.

An amniocentesis is a similar test to CVS, but it typically happens anywhere from week 13 through the last trimester of pregnancy. It can tell you whether the fetus has a host of disorders such as Down syndrome, cystic fibrosis, hemophilia, Tay-Sachs, sickle-cell anemia, toxoplasmosis, fifth disease, or cytomegalovirus. It can also confirm, later in the pregnancy, whether the baby's lungs are fully mature if a premature delivery is necessary.

The amnio tests a sample of amniotic fluid taken from the uterus through an injection through the stomach. Ultrasound is used to guide the needle to the right spot. The test can be both daunting and reassuring.

"I had the amnio, and even though I spent 23-plus years of my life on syringes, the length of the syringe totally scared me," said Erin Argueta. "But I was *so* relieved when the tests showed healthy babies."

A little knowledge can go a long way, too.

"If a CVS or amnio is recommended or desired, the procedure itself is quick and the results can be reassuring—even though the thought of the test itself can be overwhelming to some patients, especially if it is not explained thoroughly," said Dr. Tamara Takoudes.

The Fetal Echo: Scan to Your Heart's Content

For some mothers-to-be, diabetes means their developing child will undergo a fetal echocardiogram to ensure that the baby's heart has developed right and is functioning normally. This is a detailed ultrasound that focuses on the heart, and it typically takes place at a children's hospital or another facility with a pediatric cardiologist. I went to the hospital where I was first diagnosed with type 1 as a child to have my son's fetal echo at 20 weeks in utero. It was a triumphant homecoming to return there for this reason so many years later—like I'd thrived despite living with diabetes for so many years. My kid's heart test was fine, but because he moved so much during the test, the doc couldn't get the clearest look at every part of the heart. I had to return and finally got a normal test result a few weeks later.

"I had a fetal echocardiogram, which revealed a small hole in the baby's heart," said Anna Tang Norton. "I was assured it was negligible and would probably close up before I finished my pregnancy. Either way, they would do a scan on the baby's heart upon delivery to check on it. They did and found nothing abnormal."

The technology available today to be able to see something like a fetal heart thumping is pretty amazing. "It was the coolest thing to see my baby's heart pumping through all her chambers, for both my pregnancies," said Abby Nagel. "I was thrilled that both babies' hearts were completely normal with no issues."

Nonstress Tests

Nonstress tests (NSTs) usually become a regular, ongoing part of pregnancy with diabetes. The NST entails sitting down or reclining while a fetal monitor is strapped to your belly to follow the baby's movement and heart rate; it's also an indirect way to see how the placenta is functioning. The test can last a good 40 minutes, and if there's a measurement that isn't considered normal (such as a temporary deceleration of the heart rate), the test can last even longer. For someone with a well-controlled pregnancy with diabetes without high blood pressure, the NSTs begin around week 32. They typically start out weekly, and around weeks 35 to 36 they become twice-weekly tests. Sometimes you may be asked to drink cold water or to lie on your side instead of reclining on your back. Sometimes an instrument may be used to give your baby a reason to move or react to sound.

There are pros and cons to these tests. Like the many doctor's visits, the extra NSTs can be reassuring and a nice excuse to chill and read a back issue of *Us* magazine. On the flip side, these tests take up a lot of time, particularly when you don't have anything good to read or would honestly rather be doing something else—particularly without a monitor strapped to your belly. Despite their name, the NSTs can become a source of stress for one reason or another, including producing false positives. Talk to your doctor if you have concerns about the tests, the frequency, or the results. Here's what some women had to say:

- "I have mixed feelings about NSTs," said Sasha Boak Kelly. "They seemed kind of arbitrary, and my first daughter became an emergency c-section due to an irregular pattern. I am not sure that was required."

- "It was nice to have a valid excuse to just sit there and do nothing, and it was great to hear my baby's heartbeat," said Alycia Green. "My experience with them was fine, but it became a hassle to find the time to go. It started out as once a week, but then for the last two months I was supposed to be going twice a week. The hospital I went to had some really great techs and nurses, but every single time I went I had to go through a ton of questions, which took a long time."

- "I did not care for having the NSTs," said Joy McCarren. "We have independent insurance that has no maternity coverage, so for every $500 test, we paid on our own. Our doctor agreed to once a week instead of the standard two. My baby was very active, though, so I always did kick counts at home. I never felt the NSTs were useful, as things were always pretty typical. If there really was a problem, what would guarantee [that the problem wouldn't] start right after the test or [during the period] in between the scheduled tests? They just didn't seem justified to me. Some of that may be due to the fact that I'd kept myself under very tight control, so I wasn't overly worried that something would go wrong with the baby."

Going on Bed Rest

At any point in your pregnancy, possibly after you've started doing NSTs, you may learn that you need to rest by staying in bed (or on the couch). Bed rest is prescribed as a way to prevent premature labor or to help a pregnancy complicated by pre-eclampsia (high blood pressure and protein-filled urine that hit all at once) or other problems.

Bed rest can take many forms—from being told to lie still for a certain number of hours a day, to modified bed rest (no office work, driving, or household tasks), to strict bed rest at home (where you need to lie down most of the time), to going to the hospital (where you'll likely get medication to halt pre-term labor).

Some experts think that bed rest does more harm than good. Judith Maloni, PhD, RN, FAAN, a professor of nursing and a pregnancy researcher at Case Western Reserve University in Cleveland, Ohio, who focuses on the side effects of bed rest and preterm birth, believes that there is no medical reason for a women to take to her bed.[3]

"In a review of the existing evidence available internationally, there's currently no evidence to support going on bed rest," she said. "There is evidence that it is not effective and that it causes adverse side effects to the mother." These side effects include depression, muscle weakness, decreased physical fitness, and poor exercise tolerance. "If you are told you should go on bed rest, seek advice from a perinatologist [a doctor who specializes in complications during pregnancy]," she said. A second opinion from an expert in high-risk pregnancy can advise you whether the perceived benefit of bed rest is greater than the potential risks. Keep in mind, too, that going on bed rest means you won't be able to exercise or use any kind of activity to maintain your blood sugars. Your endocrinologist will provide specific instructions, but you'll likely have to increase your insulin a lot to maintain tight blood sugar numbers.

For more information about bed rest, including tips on how to cope, see Maloni's "Pregnancy Bed Rest" website at http://fpb.case.edu/Bedrest and other websites listed in the Resources section.

"In my first pregnancy I started my nonstress tests in my eighth month and failed most of them," said Abby Nagel. "In fact, I had to go to the hospital to get IV fluids to successfully stop contractions after one set of tests. On the advice of my OB/GYN, I ended up on bed rest by mid-month. I had a pretty demanding job—commuting everyday—and using public transportation had taken its toll. It was hard laying on the couch with the laptop in my lap and the phone glued to my ear for conference calls. My husband, who worked from home, would drive me into Manhattan for my nonstress tests and then take me home. It was stressful. With my second pregnancy, I was also seeing a perinatologist who tracked everything and where I did twice-a-week nonstress tests. There were a few times that I was sent over to the hospital to monitor contractions, but I was much better prepared this time. I was not surprised when I was ordered on bed rest at the beginning of my eighth month. With both pregnancies, I delivered early—the first at 34 weeks and the second at 35 weeks. Both girls were healthy and fine."

Kathryn, because of her twins' prenatal twin-to-twin transfusion syndrome, was on modified bed rest from week 17 until week 29, when she went on hospital bed rest for three weeks. "When I went on hospital bed rest, the nurses did NSTs three times a day. It was always interesting, and after a while, I could find the babies more easily than the nurses or techs," she said.

Her bed rest resulted in tender spots on her hips, and she wore her pump sites away from that area. "I wore it in a love handle on my back during delivery so it was out of the surgeon's way," she said.

While at home, Kathryn did what she could. "I could leave the house once a day," she said. "I went out for lunch and to the doctor's office, and that was it. I quit driving when I couldn't fit behind the wheel anymore. I could sit instead of lay, so I watched a lot of bad TV and sat at the computer. I was a grad student at the time, and I could do some of my research from home."

Once she entered the hospital for bed rest, Kathryn said, the toughest thing was working with the hospital's perceptions of what a person with diabetes should eat. "They couldn't understand that while I was diabetic, I had to eat more than what was on the typical diabetic diet [because of the twin pregnancy]. My husband would bring me food like hard-boiled eggs, salsa, and chips. I had to get the head nutritionist of the hospital to talk to my endocrinologist so they would understand what I needed to eat."

Biophysical Profile

Biophysical profiles, which are often combined with NSTs, measure such things as how the baby breathes, moves, and flexes its muscles (usually a finger flex rather than a bicep curl) in utero, as well as the amount of amniotic fluid you are carrying.

Your Eyes

As the eyes are affected by fluctuating blood sugars, you'll likely need to see an ophthalmologist who knows diabetic eye problems to make sure your eyes and vision don't worsen during pregnancy. If you don't have pre-existing eye concerns, you may see the eye doc only once a trimester. If you already have the beginnings, or beyond, of retinopathy or other eye issues, you'll probably see the eye doc more often because the hormonal changes during pregnancy can cause the eyes to change quickly.[4] It's important to get treatment quickly if they do.

Retinopathy occurs when the retina (the thin lining in the back of the eye) is not receiving adequate blood flow from the normal blood vessels of the eye. This may stimulate the release of a blood vessel growth factor, which can cause abnormal blood vessels to form. These new blood vessels, which grow on the surface of the retina, are small and fragile and can bleed, causing a hemorrhage in the back of the eye. They can also cause scar tissue to form, which can lead to retinal detachment. Scarring and new vessel growth can also affect your eyesight. Another type of retinopathy is macular edema, which happens when the blood vessels in the central part of the retina leak fluid, causing swelling and decreased central vision (what you see straight in front of you).

My eyes had some retinopathy going into pregnancy, and I had one bout of laser treatment on each eye for the first time while pregnant. While most nondiabetics think of laser treatment as a way to fix nearsightedness, farsightedness, and astigmatisms, laser treatment for retinopathy involves bright lights being directed at the back of your eyes (through your pupils, which are dilated) to selectively destroy part of the retina or treat areas of leakage. "Laser treatment can be very helpful in preserving vision," said Deborah Schlossman, MD, an ophthalmologist at the Joslin Diabetes Center and an instructor at Harvard Medical School. "The most important thing is that many people with retinopathy have no symptoms at all. Treatment, if needed, is most effective in the early stages. This is why it is so important to have an eye exam early in pregnancy."

I've had laser treatment three times, and the first two treatments were during my pregnancy. Before that first time,

I was terrified. I scoured the Internet for personal accounts of laser treatment for retinopathy, and I blogged about my fears. I was most worried about losing vision, either peripherally or at night. I don't wear glasses, and I read and write for a living. My actual vision was better than normal. My A1c numbers had been admirable for a few years. However, in the early years of my living with type 1, today's technologies such as home blood sugar testing, rapid insulins, and insulin pumps either did not exist or weren't widely available. My blood sugars in those early years, considered good at the time, had clearly taken their toll on my retinas by the time I reached adulthood. Pregnancy added another variable. By that point, with about 30 years of type 1 under my belt, laser eye surgery for retinopathy was my first serious complication.

Laser treatment entails numbing the eyes with drops and dilating the pupils so that a doctor can see into the back of the eyes to treat the retinas. I have had countless eye appointments where this is standard practice, so it's nothing out of the ordinary. The difference with laser treatment is that a cold lens, similar to a contact lens, is placed over your eyeball to hold the eye open. (Interestingly, it was around this time that I was asked to sign a consent form.) I rested my head on a machine with a chin rest, and my eye doctor looked into my eyes with a device that aimed bright light directly into them. Laser treatment can involve several hundred blasts of light with each procedure.

I tend to be squeamish about having drops put in my eyes, so the experience of having bright lasers in my eyes felt, at first, like I was being tortured in some foreign prison. It never hurt, save for some minor eye strain. The doctor would stop whenever the strain picked up, and after a few moments I'd give the okay for her to continue. After that first experience, a coworker gave me suggestions about what to focus on during laser treatment: the bright lights are paparazzi flashbulbs, or the spotlight on my personal stage. For my next two treatments, I kept the "Cheryl as celebrity" mindset for the whole appointment, right down to the dark sunglasses I wore out of the office. (Dilated pupils make it hard to process light, and sunglasses cut down the glare. This is temporary and resolves itself a few hours later.)

Happily, my laser treatment has not significantly affected my peripheral or night vision, and I certainly feel safe when I drive after dark. I continue to visit my eye doctor several times a year and always hope that my most recent laser experience will be my last.

Sometimes eyes damage happens during pregnancy even with careful maintenance and tight blood sugars. Bethany Rose had been treated for retinopathy several years before getting pregnant but said that despite excellent diabetes control before and during her pregnancy, "the pregnancy-related growth hormones caused new [blood vessels to grow] in my left eye." High blood pressure eventually caused those vessels to leak into the gel-like substance that fills the eye, called the vitreous. "I ended up with a big, bloody mess in the vitreous of my left eye—right in the center of my vision."

Rose was at 36 weeks and 1 day of her pregnancy and her daughter was born by c-section that evening. "I'd had small retinal bleeds before—a dot here and there—but never anything like this. It was horrible. Five weeks later, my blood pressure is under control with medication and the blood in my eye has been dissipating. My vision is still affected considerably, but my ophthalmologist is comfortable that it is clearing up on its own, albeit slowly. I expect to have more laser treatments once it clears up a little more, to minimize the chance of more bleeds in that eye." Her daughter, after a three-week stay in the hospital's intermediate care nursery (a step down from the intensive care unit), came home healthy.

The Alternative: Working With a Midwife

Maybe your diabetes has been recently diagnosed or you've never shown signs of complications. Maybe you're really uncomfortable with being classified as a high-risk pregnancy when your A1cs are in the nondiabetic range and you are a highly motivated patient who can easily handle the calculation of insulin ratios, correction factors, basal rates, carb counting, keeping detailed blood sugar records, and more. It can take a lot of research and legwork to find a midwife, but a small percentage of women with diabetes work with midwives during their pregnancies, usually in tandem with doctors.

"I work with a perinatologist and the patient, but ultimately, it's really the client who knows more about her diabetes than anyone," said Lonnie Morris, CNM, ND, a certified nurse midwife with a doctorate in nursing. She is the founder and director of the Childbirth and Women's Wellness Center, a department of Pascack Valley Hospital in Englewood, New Jersey. "These women are managing themselves." But if women with diabetes ask whether she can manage their care, Dr. Morris defers to her perinatologist's judgment about whether she can take them on as patients. "If they have additional problems"—such as uncontrolled diabetes or pre-existing kidney or eye complications—"then they're not a candidate for midwife care."

Dr. Morris, who has worked as a midwife for 35 years, has managed a small number of women with type 1 and type 2 diabetes. Midwifery is a holistic kind of care, she said. "For the first prenatal visit, I spend 45 minutes with a new patient. I talk to them about how they eat, how they live, about vitamins, whether they should wear support hose or not. There's a lot of personal support." As a midwife, she also does tests such as the 20-week anatomical scan, the nuchal translucency test, and amniocentesis.

Each patient is different, and pre-existing diabetes does not automatically mean a woman should not carry her baby to term. "We're not setting the rules so that everyone has to have the same care," she said. "There are some diabetics who get into trouble if you let them go to term. Some patients choose to be electively sectioned, and others will sail through and can deliver at term without any problems."

To find a midwife who will work with you as a patient with pre-existing diabetes, Dr. Morris suggests looking into more collaborative practices where you see midwives working with doctors. Posting to online bulletin boards that focus on diabetes and pregnancy (see Resources) can help you connect with other women with diabetes who have worked with midwives for their own pregnancies.

Yehudit W., type 1, 31, of northern New Jersey, began working with a high-risk obstetrical group, which included visits with a maternal/fetal medicine specialist. These appointments supplemented her visits to her endocrinologist and other diabetes professionals. She enjoyed the close care she received from the endocrinology group, especially their e-mail support. But the obstetrical care did not feel right for several reasons.

"First, the practice was composed of approximately 15 different doctors, any of which could have been the one to deliver my baby," she said. "I found discrepancies between the few I met regarding labor and delivery procedures. Second, it was affiliated with a hospital that had a very high c-section rate. Third, I got the feeling that they *expected* something to be wrong (why else would I be at a high-risk practice?) even though I had a very normal pregnancy and birth."

Yehudit searched for a midwife and doula (a childbirth and labor assistant), asking friends for recommendations and talking to the instructor in a class she took on the Bradley birthing method, a form of natural childbirth. A midwife can offer a different level of prenatal care than a typical high risk obstetrician might and is trained to deliver a baby; a doula is trained to help and support the mother before, during, and after giving birth.

"I ended up switching to a midwife who was backed up by a perinatologist," she said. "It was the best decision I ever made. The midwife knew exactly what I was looking for—as natural a birth as possible. I did not realize I could even switch to a midwife with my diabetes. Initially, the midwife was hesitant to take me on, but after consulting with the two perinatologists she works with, she called to let me know that she would be willing to work together with me."

Yehudit appreciated the approach her midwife took: that birth was something natural that her body was perfectly capable of handling. "One example of this was during the end of the delivery," she recalled. "My daughter's heart rate had dropped because her umbilical cord was unknowingly around her neck. My midwife gave me every last possible chance I could to be able to push her out on my own—and it ended successfully. I would imagine that if I were to have delivered with the high-risk group, they would have jumped at the first sign of distress."

While Yehudit admitted she missed the "perks of the super-high-tech equipment, working with a midwife was the right choice for me. I was looking for a birth that only one who can see it as a natural process could assist with. The doctors I had left would have most likely approached it from a purely medical standpoint. There is, and was, so much more to it than they could really be held to understand." Her daughter was born healthy and is 9 months old.

"My advice for those looking for a midwife-assisted birth is to not give up," said Yehudit. "There are midwives that are able to and will work with diabetics. Even though I left the high-risk group, I was lucky enough to continue with my endo and her team, as I had been working together with them for a number of years already."

Clemma Muller, 34, type 1, of Minneapolis, Minnesota, has two sons, aged 4 and 1. She had her first child at a Seattle, Washington, hospital, but she and her husband wanted to do something different for their second child's arrival. "Our hospital birth was not a horror story by any means, and many women would have been completely happy with it," she said. "My husband and I experienced it as traumatic, though, because it was totally the wrong birth experience for us."

An unnecessarily medicalized birth did not appeal to Muller. "My first pregnancy went perfectly," she said. "My blood sugar control was excellent, and there were no complications. My OB wanted to induce me at 38 weeks, but I managed to hold off until 40 weeks. The induction went fine, I suppose, but I hated all the interventions and the whole hospital birth and postbirth routine. I am a statistician, and I kept reading and talking to other people about type 1 pregnancy and birth. I became convinced that my induction was not necessary."

For Muller, a pregnancy with well-controlled diabetes did not warrant a high-risk designation for the birth itself. "I know that tightly controlled, healthy type 1 women using insulin pumps are still relatively unknown to many doctors, and that we are rare in delivery rooms," she said. "So I understand why they try to apply blanket protocols that aren't always necessary. Although our pregnancies are higher risk than most nondiabetic women's, I would like to see a world in which healthy type 1 women are not treated as super-high-risk births. Neither are we low-risk births—really, I think we are somewhere in between. We are medium-risk births, and the automatic early induction or caesarean protocols in the absence of some other indication beyond simply being diabetic are not appropriate in my opinion. Automatically lumping us into a group along with the truly high-risk deliveries, like octuplets or pre-eclampsia or placenta previa, and denying us birth options like the use of water-birth tubs just isn't right."

Fueled by these beliefs, Muller searched for midwives who would work with her for her second pregnancy. She began that pregnancy with an obstetrician.

Things were going pretty well, no complications again, but this time the baby always measured large on the ultrasounds. This was true from the 20-week ultrasound on. My OB started talking about "birth options," which we know means induction/caesarean, purely based on his size.

In my case, my blood sugar control had been excellent. I knew for a fact that I had not experienced chronic sustained hyperglycemia [high blood sugars], and I did not for one second believe that my baby's size was a symptom of diabetic macrosomia. I was certain that he was simply a larger-than-average baby. The ultrasound technician who did my scans told me right up to the end that he was in perfect proportions. So I felt like I was being pushed towards a totally unnecessary c-section because my OB would not or could not look past the conventional type 1 pregnancy protocol and evaluate me as an individual.

Muller found that in her state, Minnesota, certified nurse midwives practiced at hospitals and were not allowed to care for diabetics; neither were licensed midwives. Certified professional midwives were extensively trained and were certified but chose to remain otherwise unlicensed so that they were not bound by the same restraints as other midwives. "I found two women who agreed to work together for us—one had been delivering babies for nearly 30 years. They did ask me to continue to receive extra ultrasound monitoring through nonstress tests and biophysical profiles, to which I agreed because I did want that extra assurance that I wasn't developing any complications. The only thing I was worried about was that the placenta would start to fail."

Muller continued to see her obstetrician, but she did not divulge her plan to work with two midwives and prepared to deliver her child at home. "That felt icky, because my OB had been very supportive and accommodating throughout the process, but it's what I needed to do to get the birth I was convinced was the healthiest and lowest risk for me and my baby," she said.

She went into labor just past 38 weeks, after preparing herself to refuse her obstetrician's induction up to 41 weeks, and labored at home with her husband, sister, parents, and toddler son present, along with a doula, two midwives, and one apprentice. "It was quite the party," she said. "We had a birth tub set up in our bedroom, and my son was born in the water after only four hours of hard labor and pushing. He did get a little stuck, and my midwife was right on it. It wasn't shoulder dystocia, but she used a maneuver to get him out and everything was fine. She even called me the next day to debrief, and to assure me that he did not get stuck because of anything related to my diabetes. In her words,

I am 'narrow,' and at 8¾ pounds, he had a tight squeeze to get out. It was a minor and common complication that was easily resolved."

Muller is convinced that the experience was the best for her and her family. "Let me tell you how wonderful the home birth was compared to our hospital experience in Seattle," she said. "It's the difference between a medical team hovering over you, waiting for the disaster they are sure is about to happen, and a birth team that is calm and supportive, expecting everything to go right but prepared in case anything goes wrong. We did not have a backup doctor. If we had to transfer to the hospital, we were just going to show up and take whoever was on call. Our thinking was that a transfer would probably mean I needed a c-section, and in that case, we weren't going to be picky about who did it. I did write up a depressing birth plan that focused on all the bad things that could have happened, because we only expected to be at the hospital if something went wrong."

Luckily for Muller, everything went right. She and her husband managed her blood sugars on their own during the birth, testing every 15 to 30 minutes once she hit hard labor, and she wore an insulin pump throughout. Planning a home birth with a midwife isn't for everyone, she said. "For a type 1, I think there are some special criteria. I think you need to have *no* complications, especially *no* vascular complications. You need to have excellent glucose control throughout your pregnancy. I think it helps a lot if you have already given birth, so you know how to manage your own insulin during labor and delivery, because your midwife certainly won't know how to do that. Any home birth midwife should know how to watch for low blood sugar symptoms in the baby, though, and know how to treat them if they appear. I also think it's important to have some extra monitoring during the pregnancy to ensure that everything is going well, and especially that the placenta appears to be functioning normally. Ideally, you could find a care provider who would do this while knowing that you plan to do a home birth, but that didn't work out for us."

After her second son was born at home, Muller called to cancel her next obstetrician's appointment and simply told the receptionist she had had the baby at home. "I was afraid that if I had told my OB what I was planning she would have dropped me as a patient, and I didn't have time to find another provider who would give me the monitoring while knowing what I was planning." Her obstetrician never contacted her after she left the message.

If she were planning another pregnancy, Muller said, she would start with a list of all her insurance-approved obstetricians and perinatologists and contact each one, explaining that she wanted to work with someone who would provide third-trimester ultrasound monitoring for a type 1 patient planning a home birth. "Only if all of them refused would I work with a provider who didn't know my plans," she said.

However, it is very important to know that, as a woman with type 1 or type 2, choosing to work with a midwife and/or plan for a home birth is an alternative to standard medical practice for women with diabetes. It could be incredibly risky if you or your baby developed any kind of life-threatening complication that a midwife could not handle. Even if your blood sugars are fantastic and your pregnancy has had no problems at all, things sometimes happen. It is not for all—or even most—pregnant women with diabetes.

Muller herself agrees that a home birth isn't without potential danger. "No one can promise a good outcome either way," she said. "I was clear that it was all about trading one set of risks for another— that's the statistician in me. I also fully believe that with a good midwife, most complications won't have different outcomes at home than they would in the hospital. I was very confident that we had much better chances of a healthy nonintervention birth if we were at home."

Final Testing Tidbits

Your pregnancy may be punctuated by test after test and visit after visit, or you may be able to work with a provider with a less intensive approach. The most important thing is that you feel you are getting the best medical attention and care for yourself and your child throughout every stage of pregnancy. Be aware of the potential for increased risks for someone with your particular health history and of why testing is recommended. Question authority if you don't understand why a particular test is being done, how the test results have been interpreted, or what the ramifications are of any results that aren't considered normal. And if you decide to forgo some tests for any reason, talk to your doctor to ensure you are making a fully informed decision. Above all, may your pregnancy be filled with boringly normal test results, hassle-free appointments, and the excitement of knowing that your baby is thriving within you.

The Second and Third Trimesters: Things Keep Growing and Growing

5

In the Thick of It

Several months in, and things keep happening. Not only are the typical pregnancy changes taking place (You go! With your stretchy waistbands and flattering empire tops!), but the diabetes is affecting things, too. Fluctuating hormones, insulin resistance, and extra weight mean that life with diabetes will probably change all the time. Your body will become more resistant to the insulin you take, which is a normal part of any pregnancy, and you'll typically see your requirements ballooning after you get into the latter half of your second trimester. It can freak you out to see that you need so much more insulin than you needed before your pregnancy. Does it make sense to alter your diet further? And what's the deal with exercising now?

What Blood Sugars Typically Do Each Trimester

Like everything else with diabetes, your experience may differ, but typically blood sugar control varies trimester by trimester, week by week, and even day by day. According to the book *Think Like a Pancreas* by Gary Scheiner, MS, CDE, insulin requirements start dropping around week 6, dip to their lowest around weeks 9 through 11, and gradually zip up from week 12 back toward where they were before conceiving by week 16. It's unclear what causes this pattern, though it may be related, in part, to morning sickness, according to Dr. Florence Brown. After week 16, the body starts producing a cocktail of pregnancy hormones that cause insulin resistance; from then, insulin needs steadily increase up to week 36, after which they level off or even slightly decrease until delivery. "At 36 weeks, the placenta stops growing and the hormones it makes stabilize. Sometimes the insulin requirements decrease in the last three to four weeks of pregnancy, as the fetus siphons off increasing amounts of glucose," said Dr. Brown.

This means you'll need to take more insulin—sometimes double or triple (or even more) the amount you took before your pregnancy—until you give birth. After your baby and placenta are out, your insulin needs plummet. Sometimes, a day or two after delivering you might not use as much insulin as you required before your pregnancy—or any at all.

"I draw an analogy to a log flume ride at an amusement park," said Scheiner, who is the owner and clinical director of Integrated Diabetes Services, an organization that helps people manage their diabetes better. "The boat dips a bit when you first get in, then gets on the conveyor belt going up for a while, settles a bit, then takes the big plunge, dipping below surface level momentarily, before leveling off again."

Typical insulin requirements during pregnancy

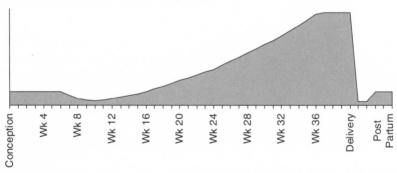

Source: Reprinted with permission from *Think Like a Pancreas: A Practical Guide to Managing Diabetes With Insulin*, Gary Scheiner, © 2004 Marlowe & Company, New York, New York.

The First Trimester

Low blood sugars can happen a lot during the first trimester, in part from trying to maintain such tight premeal ranges and because of how the body reacts during this phase of pregnancy. You may experience hypoglycemia unawareness, which is when you don't feel the symptoms of a low blood sugar or until it is much lower than where you typically feel them.

"My blood sugars dropped" at this time, said Erin Argueta. "I ran 15, 20, 30 mg/dL [at times] with each pregnancy and had to work very hard to keep myself stable. I knew the EMS technicians by name, too. They would show up and say 'Oh, it's you again?' Then they would ask what my sugar was. I remember one time telling a technician that my blood reading was 15 mg/dL, and he said, 'Wow, and you're still talking?'"

Of course, such extremely low blood sugars (and visits from emergency medical technicians) are hopefully isolated (or unheard of) incidents, not everyday events. But seeing lower numbers regularly means you must carry, or be able to find quickly, fast-acting forms of sugar and your meter to confirm what your numbers are. Carrying a cell phone can be crucial if you're alone and need to summon help fast. You might also want to get a glucagon kit, a prescription-only syringe of the hormone glucagon, which quickly raises the blood sugar by alerting the liver to release stored amounts of sugar into the blood. (This is how a nondiabetic person's body regulates itself against lows.) The kit is typically used when a person is so low she can't treat herself or refuses treatment. (If glucagon needs to be taken, it is a good idea to call 911.) However, if you're testing your blood sugar frequently—up to 10 to 20 times a day—or are using a CGM accurately, it's likely you will never go so low as to need a glucagon shot. If you are incapacitated, someone nearby needs to be able to recognize that you're low (and not passed out from too much alcohol, for example) and know how to give the injection.

"The first trimester, I did have quite a few bad low sugars," said Bronwyn Florens. "I drank a fair amount of fruit juice when I was low. However, I also needed my husband to help me at times. I went comatose more than once. If my sugars went high, I just took more insulin and monitored it myself. The doctors were not terribly worried about the occasional high level, so I learned to relax a bit. It was seldom they were very high."

Hypoglycemic episodes are common whether you are on multiple daily injections or an insulin pump, but fine-tuning can be tougher on shots alone. "I'm not on a pump, because where I live, only small children are treated with the pump," said Piret Joab, 28, type 1, of Tallinn, Estonia. She is 17 weeks into her first pregnancy. "I've been fighting with lows that started around week 6 and are still around at week 17. I have hypos daily and treating them means too-high sugars afterwards. I have to get my sugar up before I go to sleep; otherwise it will be too low in the morning. I'm constantly stressed about the fluctuations in my blood sugars, but I keep repeating to myself that the more I test, the safer the pregnancy."

Once again, a CGM can be very helpful in catching lows at, say, 60 instead of 30 mg/dL. And if you are starting to go low, treat it immediately. Even if you're lying in bed all tucked in and cozy, you're reading something fascinating, or you're running errands and really want to get to the post office before it closes, take care of the low as soon as you feel it. Treating earlier means you are less likely to go *really* low and feel worse, possibly requiring someone else's help ... or that glucagon shot.

"To manage bad lows—and there were many—I resorted to the usual juice and carbs; I also used the temporary basal setting on my insulin pump to lower my insulin until my blood sugar came back up," said Suzie Won, 38, type 1, of Huntington Beach, California. Her daughter is 15 months old. "It seemed to take longer to bring lower blood sugars back to normal when I was pregnant. I also found that drinking skim milk was a good alternative to juice for raising blood sugars gradually so that I wouldn't spike high. I also used the square wave bolus, as I noticed that food elevated my blood sugars differently when I was pregnant." The square wave—also known as the extended or combo bolus on pumps from different manufacturers—is a setting that allows you to take insulin over an extended period of time rather than all at once. It's helpful for food that raises your numbers slowly, such as meals or items with a lot of protein and/or fat.

Not everyone goes low during the first trimester. Christi Tipton, 41, type 2, of Jamestown, Tennessee, is 38 weeks into her current pregnancy and has an adopted daughter who is 3. "In my first trimester, when I found out I was pregnant, I had a significant respiratory infection and a high fever for more than 10 days," said Tipton. "My blood sugar was high—in the upper 100s and occasionally low 200s—often. I was put on progesterone supplements [a hormone that helps support an early pregnancy and helps prevent early miscarriage] and this added to the challenge of controlling my blood sugar." She was sick twice more during her first trimester, and those episodes also raised her numbers. Tipton took "a lot of correction boluses, but unfortunately, the sugars would take a while to come down," she said. "It was very unnerving to know the risks associated with high blood sugar in the first trimester and be unable to control them the way I was accustomed to doing. Even still, with all the highs I was having, my A1c did come out within normal limits."

The Second Trimester

Once the second trimester begins, insulin needs—like your belly—typically start to swell. This can be a surprise or just another twist on the wild ride that is pregnancy with diabetes. "I knew that was going to happen," said Shawna Trupiano, 34, type 1, of Avondale, Arizona. Her two sons are 4 years old and 6 months. "As long as the baby was growing properly and my blood sugars were in the range—mostly—where my team wanted them, I took it as part of diabetic pregnancy."

Dealing with your body's need for more insulin means that you're more likely to see higher numbers, which lets you know that you need to up the amounts you take. Seeing such highs can be annoying. "I didn't feel very frustrated about having to take more insulin as much as having to constantly be dealing with elevated blood sugars," said Josée Renaud. "I just wanted to find the solution to get rid of the high blood sugars as fast as possible." And "rage bolusing," as Kerri Morrone Sparling called it—taking an uncalculated amount of insulin to correct a high blood sugar, particularly one that doesn't respond to prior correction boluses—can be common. "I treat highs—in the 200s—aggressively because I get angry about them," said Suzanne Hagen, 35, type 1, of Northbrook, Illinois. She is 24 weeks into her first pregnancy.

Even if you know intellectually that what is happening is normal during pregnancy, it can be tough to see insulin needs increase so dramatically. "I took an incredible amount of insulin—at least a couple hundred units total each day at the very end of my pregnancy," said Elizabeth "Bjay" Woolley. "I felt really guilty. I don't like to take medications of any kind, and it was tough for me to put so much in my body. I asked my endocrinologist about it, and he said 'Yes, it's a lot,' but he had other patients who took a lot more. I felt a little better after that. It was a big relief when the pregnancy was over and my insulin needs went down."

The jump can seem almost irresponsible to some people. When not pregnant, when you eat the appropriate amount of food to maintain a healthy body weight, you need whatever amount of insulin keeps your blood sugar numbers in a healthy range. Eat more than your body needs, and take more insulin to cover the effect on your blood sugars, and that extra food stays on your body as excess weight, as it does for anyone without diabetes who overeats. This is why the idea that "insulin makes you fat" circulates among those who don't understand the intricacies of life with diabetes, particularly insulin-dependent diabetes. Again, if your body needs extra insulin to maintain your blood sugar control, take whatever you need to take. If your body doesn't need the food, it stores it as fat. If your body needs it—particularly while you're pregnant—you won't gain excess weight. You'll gain some weight as a *normal and healthy* part of pregnancy, but that weight should come off after you give birth.

"My response was a surprise to me," said Yehudit W. "I knew that people who were overweight tend to need more insulin. Being a health nut, I didn't want that stigma. In response, I retrained myself to ignore that and focused on obtaining stellar blood sugars, no matter how much insulin it took. I strived to do everything possible to maintain the range of blood sugars for a healthy pregnancy."

The whatever-it-takes approach is probably the sanest, and using all the tools available to you can make things easier to handle and to respond to quickly. "With input from my medical team, my ratios changed about every two weeks or more often if needed," said Kathryn. "No big deal, because I was told to expect this. I just had to use a calculator sometimes because math in my head wasn't working so well, being pregnant! Also, I was so glad I had an insulin pump at this point. Seriously, I was eating little bits of food all day and practically all night long. Taking that many shots would have been a pain in the tush, literally. Even though I had to change my site daily because of the amount of insulin I was taking, it was still only one needle per day, instead of 20 little shots."

The insulin pump is a precise way to see how much insulin you are taking: most pumps show your total daily dose. "I noticed I was going through more insulin as I progressed in pregnancy, and gained a modest amount of weight," said Anna Tang Norton. "I also noticed I was changing infusion sites every two days instead of every three." (An infusion site is where the tiny plastic tube that transfers insulin from your pump into your body is inserted under the skin.)

Keeping a current prescription for syringes isn't a bad idea if you're using a pump full time. I used to take some meal insulin doses by syringe so that I could keep my infusion sets in longer—using the pump more for underlying basal rates. I did this in the third trimester particularly, when meal insulin doses were gigantic. Using a syringe can also get insulin into your body quickly if you're noticing high blood sugars that aren't responding to correction—or rage—boluses. Before changing an infusion set, you can inject the insulin and then investigate whether your infusion set has gone bad or is blocked. Blockage can cause blood sugars to read higher if the insulin isn't being absorbed effectively or at all. Typically, an infusion set lasts about three days under the skin. After that, it should be changed to avoid infection or irritation at the site; however, some of us have been known to keep the set in the body longer if blood sugar numbers appear to be stable and the site still looks good—meaning it isn't inflamed, sore, tender, or itchy. As always, your experience may be different.

On the flip side, lows can still happen despite insulin resistance. "In my second trimester, I began to have some more significant hypoglycemia episodes," said Christi Tipton. "My hypoglycemia awareness changed dramatically. Instead of my usual signs when I was in the low 70s or upper 60s, I had virtually none until I was in the low 50s. It became common for me to check my blood sugar simply because I was feeling suddenly tired, or a little agitated, or grumpy [a symptom Tipton hadn't associated with hypoglycemia before], and I would discover that my blood sugar was in the 50s."

For some, settling into pregnancy can bring predictability and better numbers. "My sugars got tighter during my second trimester," said Kathryn. "I had tighter control. I think I just got better at anticipating what was going on with my body in relationship to the food I ate and activity level I had that day."

The Third Trimester

By the third trimester, you may be in touch with your doctor's office even more frequently. With insulin resistance typically hitting even harder now, your regimen can require many adjustments, with phone calls, faxes, and visits with your endocrinologist and CDE to fine-tune anything from insulin-to-carb ratios, to basal rates for pump users, to diet.

"I adjusted my ratios one meal at a time and one day at a time," said Shawna Trupiano. "If my one and two hour postprandial [after-meal] numbers were not where my team and I wanted them, then my team left it up to me to tweak my ratios a little at a time, as I would see the results first. Then, as I switched ratios, I sent my team a fax that said the previous ratio and a new ratio, along with a time and date. They seemed to change about once every three days. It was annoying sometimes to have all of a sudden something not working that worked yesterday, but I knew that it would change, also."

For those who can adjust their own insulin and carb ratios effectively, all the visits might seem, again, extraneous. Of course, while no one knows your diabetes as well as you do, doctors tend to see many more patients who are not as motivated and aware about their diabetes as you might be. So if you happen to be a superstar patient, consider yourself the exception not the rule.

"Each person is different, and some love having their doctors being in constant contact and control of their diabetes management," said Joy McCarren. "I am not like that, and because we have no maternity coverage, I would get very frustrated with my doctors when they expected to see me 'just because' I was diabetic. My best advice for handling the visits and the extra blood sugar logging is to just take it one day at a time. As long as you know you are doing the best you possibly can, don't let any of your doctors make you feel bad for not logging some of your blood sugars or for asking for your appointments to be spaced a little farther apart. It is definitely important to be in contact with your doctors, but if you are in very tight control of your diabetes, I think there should be consideration given to the patient by the doctors. Doctors need to be willing to listen to any of our concerns about so many visits, and understand that each diabetic is different, and so is each pregnancy."

Some medical offices, either because of distance or because it works best for them, rely on technology more than others. "I live in a small town, and my diabetes team is approximately six hours away from me," said Josée Renaud. "So I am in contact with my nurse every week via e-mail, and she helps me make adjustments to my insulin dosages."

If you can download blood sugar readings or insulin doses from your meter, pump, or CGM, ask whether your doctor wants those logs only or whether she's more old school and prefers to see handwritten records that include the kind and amount of food eaten as well as blood glucose and insulin information.

Of course, highs and lows will likely continue to happen— hopefully occasionally rather than frequently—throughout the third trimester. "There were times when I became very hypoglycemic, but I would just take some glucose tablets and wait," said Alycia Green. "Hypoglycemia is no fun at all, but for it to happen during pregnancy—that just put extra fright into me. I was constantly paranoid about what effects that might have on my child." Again, as a reminder from Chapter 1, lows are only a problem for your functioning and well-being; the risk of lows possibly affecting your baby's development increase if you are running your blood sugars, on average, at 86 mg/dL—which corresponds to a 4.6 percent A1c—or lower.

Treating highs in the third trimester can be tougher than before because insulin resistance is so persistent. It can be helpful to have a few techniques to try in case one option doesn't work as well as it once did. "During my third trimester, I had more insulin resistance and had to increase my basals," said Lindsay Gopin. "For highs, I would always try to exercise—walk—for 20 minutes to get my sugars down more quickly."

Others use a technique called the super bolus, which was pioneered by John Walsh, PA, CDE, coauthor with Ruth Roberts of the book *Pumping Insulin: Everything You Need for Success on a Smart Insulin Pump*.[1] The super bolus is a way for insulin pump users to take extra insulin immediately by adding a percentage of the future basal delivery to the bolus before eating a high-carb meal; this technique helps prevent the postmeal blood sugar spike from going quite as high.

It can require some trial and error, but essentially it means taking a certain percentage of the amount of basal insulin you would take over the next three hours and adding it to whatever you would typically bolus for that meal. (Walsh said he would typically shift no more than 80 percent of the basal rate into a super bolus but you may fnd a different percentage, either lower or higher, works best for you.) You then set a temporary basal rate over that three-hour period of the remaining percentage of your typical basal rate per hour (20 percent if you take 80 percent for the super bolus, using Walsh's maximum as an example). The early delivery of most of the basal insulin, combined with the bolus insulin, speeds up the insulin's effect, and the temporary basal reduction prevents you from going too low and having an insulin reaction.

As an example, if you are planning to eat a meal with 50 grams of carbs and typically use an insulin ratio of 1 unit of insulin to 10 grams of carbs, you count 5 units of insulin for the food alone. If your basal rate is 1 unit per hour, over three hours your insulin pump would give you 3 units of insulin. With the super bolus, you take 80 percent of those 3 units (which is 2.4 units) up front, along with the 5 units for the meal. That is, you take 7.4 units of insulin for the meal and 20 percent of your normal basal rate over the next three hours, and your blood sugar should hopefully rise less than it would if you took your insulin the conventional way. (It's a lot of math, but most insulin pumps can be programmed to do the number crunching for you.)

Another technique to try is taking your insulin 10 to 15 minutes before you eat (provided you're above 70 mg/dL when you start and know your blood sugar isn't dropping quickly). "This will improve the timing of insulin action so that it matches the absorption of the meal glucose," said Dr. Florence Brown. She also recommends increasing your insulin-to-carb ratio to provide an adequate bolus to cover the rise in blood sugar one to two hours after you eat, along with reducing your basal rates to prevent low blood glucose three to four hours after the meal.

Toward the final weeks of pregnancy, it's common to see insulin needs stabilize. "One thing I see very often in the online pregnancy groups is that around weeks 34 through 36, the insulin resistance goes down and there are a lot of lows," said Allison Herschede. "Every mom freaks out when this happens and thinks the placenta is failing. I asked my perinatologist about this and he said that while they used to think that this signified placental deterioration, they now know better. He said it is completely normal, but did check the placenta and blood flow on an ultrasound, which made me feel better." This is the equivalent of doing a biophysical profile to examine the status of the placenta.

Tips to Help You Test More Frequently

If you're not using a CGM—or even if you are—testing frequently helps you know what your blood sugars are doing on a regular basis. For some people, it's just automatic to be testing before meals, one to two hours after a meal, before bed, before driving, before and after exercise, in the middle of the night, whenever they feel low, and any other time it feels right to test. For others, different things can motivate and remind them that it's time to check the sugars again:

- "I put myself on a rigid schedule of testing as soon as I woke up, before every meal and one hour after every meal, before I went to bed, and I set my alarm at 3 a.m. every night to test," said Abby Nagel. "It was brutal, but kept my sugars in check."

- "Knowing that your actions are making a direct impact on the health of your baby is a strong motivator," said Suzie Won. "It's normal to feel scared or nervous if you haven't felt the baby kick or if you occasionally run a high blood sugar. That's why I felt it was important to use the CGM, even though at the time, I had to pay out of pocket."

- "I am on the CGM, so I test to calibrate it about three times daily," said Josée Renaud. "I started the system at week 10 of my pregnancy and before then, I tested about 15 times a day, including twice during the night. Always have your blood glucose machine close by with a log book to insert the results right away."

- "I was testing eight times a day: upon waking, before meals, two hours after meals, and before bed, in addition to anytime I felt 'off,'" said Alycia Green. "It is easy enough to remember to test before meals and when you wake up, but it takes diligence to remember to do it two hours after. I usually ate meals around the same time every day, so I just set an alarm on my cell phone to notify me two hours after those standard meal times."

- "Set reminders on your pump if you have that option," said Kathryn. "I didn't on my pregnancy pump, but I do on the one I have now. *Wow*, that function would have been really helpful. Otherwise, get a watch with an alarm and use the alarm to remind you."

- "Keep your machine with you wherever you go," said Bronwyn Florens. "If I thought of my baby's health all the time, then it was easy to test."

- "Test every hour—just don't forget," said Lindsay Gopin.

- "The fear of birth complications helped me [test often], not that you want to be thinking about that all the time," said Sasha Boak Kelly. "I also used to set up Google e-mail reminders to send me instant popup messages on my computer screen at work to say TEST TEST. It worked. As a last ditch, I would set alarms on my insulin pump, which would sound an alarm that was annoying enough to make me pay attention.

- "I tested mine obsessively," said Amy Eddy. "If you want to have a healthy baby, you just have to remember to do it frequently. It's all self-discipline. The more you care, the more diligent you will be."

Keep in mind that all this stuff is truly a lot of work, even if it takes only a minute or less to do a test. Making sure that your meter is well stocked with strips and extra lancets, that your prescriptions are adequate for the number of tests you are doing, and that the strips arrive on time if you fill your prescriptions by mail, is a lot to remember. Don't forget about logging the results, and spending the mental energy to note the patterns and trends in your blood sugar readings. This all takes up valuable brain space, that, honestly, most people don't have to worry about. Do whatever it takes to make testing easier for you. The test strip containers that I use come with 25 strips in a package, but it's easy to run through a container if you are testing so many times a day. I would put 50 strips into one container so that I wouldn't run out of strips as quickly, particularly if I was away from my home stash. As mentioned in Chapter 1, I use one meter, but some people find it easier to test if they keep meters in several locations, such as at work, at home, and in the car. If your insurance company hassles you for testing more frequently, try to have your doctor or her office argue with them on your behalf. An insurance company cannot practice medicine. If your doctor says it is medically necessary for you to test your blood sugar more times a day than the insurance company thinks you should, your doctor's opinion should overrule whatever song and dance the insurance company is trying to give you. Push your doctor's office to work it out with the insurance company on your behalf if you need to.

How to Deal With Testing Results

It's one thing to remember to test all the time; it's another to know what to do with all the information. Yes, the more you know, the healthier you can be, but sometimes you can drown in a sea of data. Here are a few life preservers to help you navigate without too much frustration:

- **Don't declutter yet.** "Keep a folder to organize all your lab tests and results," said Suzie Won. Having everything in one place, including blood sugar logs, records of insulin doses, and notes from prior appointments, makes it easier to figure out what's going on with you, particularly if you have follow-up questions about lab results, changing ratios, or just how your sugars look day by day. "Keep a notebook that you take to every appointment with you," said Kathryn. "Make sure what you are understanding from each of the docs makes sense, and that everyone on your medical team is communicating well among each other and with you."

- **Don't sweat the highs too much.** I know, easier said than done. But as mentioned earlier, we all have high blood sugars—that's what living with diabetes means. The key is to bring them down as quickly and safely as possible, and to focus on making sure they don't happen frequently. "I worked extremely hard keeping my sugars down," said Amy Eddy. "When I did get the occasional high, I freaked out and worried that I killed my baby. Yeah, I was nutty like that. But the occasional high isn't going to hurt your baby—just make sure you're doing everything you can to have a healthy baby: eat right, test often, and make sure your insulin dosing schedule is effective, which can only be determined by frequent testing."

- **Fix the lows as soon as possible.** While you don't want to overtreat a low and then have to battle a high, find something you can tolerate to help treat your lows quickly. Personally, I detest glucose tabs. I think they're pricey and chalky, so I never use them. LifeSavers or juice boxes are better for me. People have their own preferences. "I have had some lows in the 30s and 40s, but nothing severe," said Suzanne Hagen. "I just treated them as I always did with juice, glucose tablets, Jelly Bellies, or candy corn—a newfound old favorite."

- **Do look at the big picture.** "I am a perfectionist, so if I had a high number, it freaked me out," said Abby Nagel. "I often had to look at my averages and see that my average was normal for a nondiabetic. That often helped me cope and not stress out."

- **Accept that blood sugar control, like pregnancy, can involve a lot of watching and waiting.** "Sometimes I'm frustrated that I can't make the changes quickly enough to respond to the patterns," said J. Davis Harte, 37, type 1, of Corvallis, Oregon. She is 31 weeks into her first pregnancy. Some people can make changes themselves a few days after noticing a pattern; others rely on their endocrinologist to make the adjustments. "I find that for me, I need to make adjustments myself, but my endo will also make changes as is necessary. It's a constant multiseated teeter-totter of variables."

- **Don't go it alone.** Once again, seek support online if you need it. Use the Resources section to find people who can relate to exactly what you are going through. "I searched pregnancy message boards where other people discussed their results," said Bronwyn Florens. "While this can make you worry more, it can also be a relief and help you interpret results based on others' reactions to their own results. It helps you realize that a large array of results can be normal, and that even when results are not completely normal, they can be acceptable." Find sites that are legit and the most helpful. "Ask your doctor for reputable sites and do not jump to conclusions based on what you read online," said Suzie Won.

- **Remember that there's more to life than dealing with diabetes.** If this is your first pregnancy, this is the last stretch of time when it'll just be you and your partner. Enjoy the time as much as you can. "Go to movies, concerts, play sports, or take up a new hobby now, because you won't have time once the baby arrives," said Suzie Won.

The Eating Thing—Revisited

As the weeks and months pass, you may find yourself in a food groove: you know what to eat so that you're satisfied, you're getting enough nutrition for two, and your blood sugars are where you want them to be.

"I had a salad with grilled shrimp almost every day with a small bag of popcorn—yummy—and my one can of Diet Coke," said Abby Nagel. "By the end of my pregnancy, the salad server at the deli I went to knew me and prepared my order before I even opened my mouth!"

Some foods are definitely more popular than others when it comes to eating while pregnant. Proteins such as eggs and cheese, healthier fats such as raw almonds, Greek yogurt, peanut butter, and other nut butters, and high-fiber carbs such as tortillas, popcorn (especially the 100-calorie bags), and oat bran can fill you up without shooting your sugars too high (or up at all). Nearly all vegetables fall into this category, too (though keep an eye on the higher-carb ones like carrots; you might think you're eating a great easy snack of baby carrots, but a full bag of them can tally more than 80 grams of carb—which necessitates a good hit of insulin). Celery dipped in peanut butter or low-fat cream cheese, sugar-free pudding, either instant or made with soy or almond milk, and sugar-free popsicles are other snack ideas. Of course, if you hate celery but love red pepper or are avoiding peanut butter because of a family history of allergy and want to substitute hummus instead, that's fine too. Whatever works.

Sometimes nausea or illness dictates what you eat, even well into the pregnancy. "I found that Slim-Fast has all the nutrients with almost half the carbs for a morning snack," said Christi Tipton. "I rely on it a lot. There are many mornings I don't eat at all before noon because of insulin resistance, but when I am very hungry or my blood sugar is low and I need to eat, Slim-Fast has been a lifesaver." (Despite how you feel, however, it is not a good idea to skip a meal because of the potential to spill ketones as a result, said Dr. Florence Brown.)

In some cases, surprising foods can both satisfy you and keep your sugars in line, provided you know exactly how much insulin to take. "Sometimes I would give in and have a Snickers candy bar that I knew was a solid 35 grams of carbs, as well as peanuts—so it wasn't all bad," said Shawna Trupiano. "That was a nice snack with a glass of cold milk to fill me up between meals. With the proper bolusing, I was able to stay a little more flatline with my blood sugars."

Speaking of flatlining, some people eliminate foods that worked fine for them before they were pregnant and swap them for new ones precisely to avoid up-and-down blood sugars:

- "I've had to switch to eating a low-carb breakfast in the morning, so I'm making friends with cottage cheese," said J. Davis Harte. "I add in some cinnamon to make it more palatable. I love eggs, but I find that it can be tricky to make the time to prepare them in the morning hurry. At other times of the day besides the morning, I seem to be able to handle eating carbs."

- "We are all individuals," said Christi Tipton. "Each of us responds our own way to foods, to meds, to stress, to pregnancy. For example, oatmeal is a food they all suggest for pregnancy, yet even the smallest amount will make my blood sugar go far too high, even with adequate insulin. And whole-grain bread can make me go far too high, too fast. I have a hard time coming back down again. Yet rice and pasta are easy foods for me, with little spike to my blood sugars. I can also enjoy watermelon and some other fruits, like apples, with little spike as well."

- "At times I was surprised by just how much more insulin I needed and how much resistance I had," said Joy McCarren. "Especially when it came to foods that I used to be able to eat, but couldn't anymore without my blood sugar going crazy. I would get frustrated, but never really guilty, because I knew that no matter how much insulin I had to take, it wasn't crossing over to the baby. But if I didn't take it, and let my sugars run high, the baby would be forced to make more of its own insulin and run the risk of complications down the road. Being able to talk to other diabetics who have been through pregnancy is very encouraging since they tend not to judge. They've been there and know just how hard a diabetic pregnancy can be."

Exercise: It's Good For You ... Except When It Isn't

Working out has a lot of well-known benefits when it's just your own body you're working, including lowering your blood sugar numbers,

How Exercise Helps You

Becoming active and exercising at least 30 minutes on most, if not all, days of the week can benefit your health in the following ways:

- Helps reduce backaches, constipation, bloating, and swelling
- Increases your energy
- Improves your mood
- Improves your posture
- Promotes muscle tone, strength, and endurance
- Helps you sleep better

Regular activity also helps keep you fit during pregnancy and may improve your ability to cope with the pain of labor. This will make it easier for you to get back in shape after the baby is born. You should not, however, exercise to lose weight while you are pregnant.

Source: American College of Obstetricians and Gynecologists. *Exercise During Pregnancy*. ACOG Patient Education Pamphlet AP119. Washington, DC: ACOG, 2003. Reprinted with permission.

keeping your heart healthy, reducing stress levels, increasing energy, and keeping excess weight gain in check. All good—so what's the difference about doing it (or starting to exercise) with a baby on board?

If you worked out regularly before getting pregnant, sticking with exercise will help you counteract the insulin increases that typically occur when you are with child. "Being active will keep you from having to raise your insulin doses as much, even during the last few months of your pregnancy," writes Sheri Colberg, PhD, the author of the *Diabetic Athlete's Handbook* and seven other books about diabetes and/or exercise (quotes reprinted with permission from Human Kinetics).[2] "Being active will also prevent excessive weight gain and keep you from getting out of shape. If you have to stop exercising during your pregnancy for any reason, expect your insulin needs to go up dramatically, both from the hormones released and from the decrease in your insulin action that will you experience from being inactive."

Carrying the extra weight of pregnancy can itself feel like a workout. "Pregnancy increases the energy costs of doing any activity, so you will be using more calories during all your activities, particularly the weight-bearing ones," writes Dr. Colberg. "Your exercise intensity will likely go down, particularly in the later stages of your pregnancy as Mother Nature takes care of your baby's health by not making it possible for you to work out as hard as normal (even if you try to)."

But if you weren't a jock beforehand, or just considered yourself a casual exerciser, is it safe to start up (again) while pregnant? It depends on your health—both before pregnancy and during. "A patient needs to be evaluated by her doctors, in terms of any diabetes complications, to determine the risks and benefits of exercising," said Jacqueline Shahar, MEd, CDE, a registered clinical exercise physiologist, and the manager of exercise physiology at the Joslin Diabetes Center.

Bodily Changes to Expect While Pregnant

Joints

The hormones produced during pregnancy cause the ligaments that support your joints to become relaxed. This makes the joints more mobile and more at risk of injury. Avoid jerky, bouncy, or high-impact motions that can increase your risk of injury.

Balance

With as much as 25–40 pounds at the end of pregnancy, extra weight in the front of your body shifts your center of gravity and places stress on joints and muscles, especially those in the pelvis and lower back. This can make you less stable, cause back pain, and make you more likely to lose your balance and fall, especially in later pregnancy.

Heart Rate

The extra weight you are carrying will make your body work harder than before you were pregnant. Exercise increases the flow of oxygen and blood to the muscles being worked and away from other parts of your body. So, it's important not to overdo it.

Source: American College of Obstetricians and Gynecologists. *Exercise During Pregnancy.* ACOG Patient Education Pamphlet AP119. Washington, DC: ACOG, 2003. Reprinted with permission.

Definitely get the go-ahead from your doctor on whether you can exercise and how much. With some medical conditions, you might be recommended to avoid exercise, said Michael See, MS, RCEP, clinical exercise physiologist at the Joslin Diabetes Center. These conditions include carrying multiples, high blood pressure, a history of pre-eclampsia, vaginal bleeding in the second or third trimesters, premature membrane rupture, a history of premature labor, premature labor itself, placenta previa (when the placenta is positioned over the cervix), incompetent cervix (when the cervix is weakened and opens prematurely), or cerclage (when the cervix is sewn closed until a few weeks before a term pregnancy). Even if you don't have any of these conditions but weren't a fitness buff before you got pregnant, don't plan to train for your first triathlon now that you're with child—be honest with yourself and your doctor about how active you were before you were pregnant.

General Guidelines for Exercise

For anyone, with diabetes or not, exercise should always be safe and beneficial. Michael See suggests the following tips:

- Try to exercise at least a half hour a day (provided you are healthy and there is no medical reason not to do so).

- Dress for fitness: wear loose and comfortable clothing and look for fabrics that will keep sweat away from your skin. Wear a bra that gives proper support and sneakers that fit well.

- Exercise in a cool and well-ventilated place. When it's hot or humid outside, find an air-conditioned or otherwise more comfortable environment to exercise in.

- Don't exercise while lying flat on your back after your first trimester.

- Hydrate: drink at least a glass (8 ounces) of water during your workout. Don't wait to be thirsty to drink water.

- After you exercise, cool down gradually. This will help you avoid feeling faint or dizzy and will keep your blood circulating properly.

"There really aren't any exercise guidelines for pregnant people with diabetes that I know of," said Dr. Sheri Colberg. "In general, the main goal of exercising with diabetes is to maintain blood sugars, however you have to do that." As a result, there's a lot of trial and error when it comes to figuring out how exercise might affect one woman with diabetes over another, and a lot depends on how active you were before getting pregnant. A runner who has completed several marathons over the years is different from a newer jogger who just did her first 5K, and both are at a different place from the woman who gets worked up from a short stroll around the block.

If you're type 2 and relatively new to insulin, know that exercise can significantly affect the absorption of insulin and can drop your blood sugars quickly. Type 1? This is probably old hat, but when you exercise, always have your glucose meter, strips, a finger-pricker, and a source of fast-acting glucose handy to treat any lows. Test before you begin each workout. If you haven't eaten recently and you're 250 mg/dL or higher, check to see whether you're spilling ketones. If you are, drink water to flush them out of your body and hold off on the exercise until you go lower and have lost the ketones entirely. If you do exercise when you're so high, your blood sugar is more likely to spiral up instead of coming down.

If you test and you're between 250 and 300 mg/dL and *don't* have ketones, and you still want to work out, consider when you last ate, when you last took insulin, and whether it is actively working in your body or its effectiveness has already peaked. If you don't have insulin actively working in your body from a recent bolus or injection, you may want to consider giving yourself a *small* amount of insulin to help kick-start your blood sugar reduction alongside the exercise (but definitely don't take as much as a typical correction if you're going to exercise afterward or you are bound to bottom out during or after your workout).

Also, keep an eye on how intense your activity is. "When numbers are high, I would not recommend vigorous activity, with or without pregnancy," said Jacqueline Shahar. This puts more stress on the body, which in turn causes hormones to alert the liver to produce even more sugar. The result? Blood sugars can go up even with more exercise. Stick to low or moderate activity and drink water to flush the sugar through the urine.

Activity levels can be based on heart rates (beats per minute) or the ratio of perceived exertion scale, said Shahar. The latter method asks you to rate how you feel during exercise and helps you figure out your tolerance for activity. "Think of a scale of 6 to 20," she said. "You want to be in the range of 11 to 13. The easy way to think of it is that you're trying to be at 110 to 130 beats per minute."

If you don't have a heart rate monitor to figure this out and don't trust yourself to know when you're working a bit harder than halfway to exhaustion (think of the low end as no effort at all and the high end as the hardest you've ever worked in your life), there's an easy way to estimate your heart rate. After you've been exercising for a few minutes, take your pulse by putting your pointer and middle finger together and holding them to the carotid artery in the front of your neck. If you find the right spot, you'll feel a pulsing as your heart beats. (You might also feel this pulse at your inner wrist). Count the beats for exactly six seconds (use a watch that counts the seconds) and add a zero to the number you get. This is your approximate heart rate in beats per minute.

Some activities are more comfortable and/or safer than others while you are pregnant. "Most of the time, it's not recommended that you do maximal or even sustained vigorous exercise when pregnant," said Dr. Sheri Colberg, in an e-mail interview. "Most of the studies have been done on animals, but they indicate that intense exercise can compromise blood flow to the fetus and may cause hyperthermia [an abnormal increase in temperature] that, if sustained, may be harmful to the fetus."

Hyperthermia can happen at other times, too. Skip exercising when it's hot and humid or if you already have a fever, said Jacqueline Shahar. And to prevent getting dehydrated, drink water before, during, and after exercise; dehydration can cause muscle cramps, high blood sugars, and heat stroke and can reduce muscle performance, she said.

Exercise doesn't always make things better. Watch out for the following problems (see box on next page) and get help right away if necessary.

Modifications You Might Make

In general, mild to moderate aerobic exercise is the most beneficial. What's safest: walking, low-impact aerobics, swimming and other water activities, stationary cycling, elliptical training, light weights, resistance bands, and yoga. What's not so safe: vigorous intense

Warning Signs

Stop exercising and call your doctor if you get any of these symptoms:

- Vaginal bleeding
- Dizziness or feeling faint
- Increased shortness of breath
- Chest pain
- Headache
- Muscle weakness
- Calf pain or swelling
- Uterine contractions
- Decreased fetal movement
- Fluid leaking from the vagina

Source: American College of Obstetricians and Gynecologists. *Exercise During Pregnancy*. ACOG Patient Education Pamphlet AP119. Washington, DC: ACOG, 2003. Reprinted with permission.

exercises such as sprinting and running, water skiing (which has the potential to force water into the vagina—not so good), any breath-holding activities, or any activities that require you to lie flat on your back (some yoga and Pilates poses). It's a good idea to avoid sports where you could fall (downhill skiing, skating, outdoor biking if you crash) or lose your balance as a result of quick directional changes (racquet sports, handball, kickboxing). And according to Michael See, sky diving and scuba diving are also generally not recommended during pregnancy, for assorted reasons.

Then again, do you *really* feel like sky or scuba diving these days? For me, just putting on a pair of socks in my third trimester felt like running a marathon. For others, it's tough enough to haul a pregnant body—with its newfound heft, swollen ankles, and aching joints—out of bed.

Regardless, when you are up for working out, do it at a comfortable pace if your endocrinologist and obstetrician have cleared you for exercise during pregnancy. Sometimes, though, pregnancy has other plans for you. If you're exhausted, achy, or really, Really, REALLY not interested in exercising right now, that's okay too. (Though a bit of mild exercise, such as a walk around the block, might actually make you feel much better as well as help your blood sugars.)

"I tried to keep active through semi-regular walking and prenatal yoga, but I did find that difficult during some of the more tiring stages of the pregnancy," said Bethany Rose. "I often just didn't feel like I had the energy. Plus, I had a lot of discomfort in my hips during the second trimester, so I had to take it easy then. It was a bit frustrating, because walking and yoga helped my hips feel better afterward, but was difficult to get started because it was uncomfortable initially."

When she was able to do yoga, Rose found it ideal because it didn't affect her diabetes control. "It was low intensity, so it didn't wreak havoc on my blood sugar, and the poses and stretches are really geared to your changing body and at the muscles that are tired from pregnancy as well as the muscles you will need to use during delivery," she said. "It's also very relaxing."

Others aspired to maintain the level of fitness they had before pregnancy. "I stayed moderately active throughout the entire pregnancy," said Anna Tang Norton. "I walked and swam mostly. I would tell others to keep moving—it definitely helps with the swelling and overall well-being. There's no reason to do anything super-strenuous, but moving is a good thing for circulation; plus, it's good to get some natural air." Amy Mercer, in her third pregnancy, found she could keep doing a modified routine. "With this pregnancy, I have continued to run the entire time," she said. "For my first two pregnancies, I stopped running as soon as I found out I was pregnant and walked for the duration of the pregnancy. This time, many years later, I've felt pretty good. I am running very slowly, stop to walk when I get tired, and I am not going too far. Most importantly, I listen to my body. It's really helped: at 28 weeks, I have only gained 22 pounds and more importantly, I am retaining my sanity!"

As mentioned earlier, for those who can keep moving and aren't exhausted, insulin requirements may be lower than expected. "I practice and teach yoga," said Suzanne Hagen. "My total daily dose of insulin was less than it was pre-pregnancy for quite a while. I guess that is normal, but it's continued for longer than the doc said it might ... it's because I'm so active. If I were sedentary, this would not be the case." While she was sluggish in her first trimester, Hagen has returned to her regular workouts, modified, now that she is well into her second trimester. "I've had to find some variations for yoga poses or simply not do some. I've altered my weightlifting routine and have had to find different ab exercises. I have also continued walking briskly and have done some hiking and a short backpacking trip, though my husband carried more of the weight that time."

Some health issues make exercise modifications a must, say exercise experts Shahar, See, and Colberg. With any exercise, there's an increase in blood pressure, so if you're already dealing with hypertension, stick with activity that won't raise the systolic (top) number of your blood pressure readings excessively such as holding your breath while lifting heavy weights. Low to moderate cardio activity should be okay, but check with your doctor. If you have nonproliferative eye issues, watch that systolic blood pressure number and keep it from rising too high; it should be 180 or lower, said Shahar. If retinopathy is proliferative (new blood vessels are growing in the back of the eyes), be careful with weightlifting and activities where your head is down—certain yoga poses, for example—and avoid "jumping or jarring activities," said Dr. Colberg. "Do not exercise during retinal hemorrhages." For neuropathy (nerve damage), if your feet are numb or painful or lack sensation, check them regularly for blisters and other traumas and be aware of balance issues. With mild kidney problems, stick with low to moderate activity that won't cause systolic blood pressure to rise. With the more serious problem of pre-eclampsia (which includes hypertension and albumin spilled in the urine), talk to your doctor about what's best, as advice can vary case by case.

Working out in water is a popular pregnancy choice, as the buoyancy can help you feel less beached whale and more sleek mermaid. "[I take an] aqua aerobics class and plan to continue for the remainder of my pregnancy," said J. Davis Harte. "Nothing feels as good to my swollen ankles as being in the water! I'm planning on adding in more water exercise classes so that I can spend more time in the pool. Walking the dogs is also a must-do activity, but sometimes my feet are just too sore and tender for walking." If you're close to a swimming area with an on-duty lifeguard and enjoy water-based exercise, take advantage of it during pregnancy. "If I had access to a swimming pool, I'd definitely use it," said Yehudit W. "It supposedly is easier to work out in, as the water distributes the extra weight of the pregnancy, and you don't feel it so much. You can still get a normal all-body workout without getting

as tired." Swimming, or any other cardio workout in water, feels wonderful on the joints because of the buoyancy, said Joslin's Michael See.

Despite the benefits, some women forgo fitness altogether. This is
often due to health restrictions, although pure exhaustion is certainly
a legit reason, too:

- "My exercise was brought to a halt as I started to swell and
  had some blood pressure issues," said Shawna Trupiano.
  "The following week, when they had not improved, I was put
  on modified bed rest until I went into labor on my own at 32
  weeks and my son was born a day later." After a short neonatal intensive care unit (NICU) stay, Trupiano's son went
  home with her, healthy, at 3 days old.

- "Right now, I barely exercise since the minute I move myself,
  I get too low blood sugar," said Piret Joab. "I only do some
  walking, with a bottle of juice."

- "I had bad round-ligament pain from the beginning, so I
  didn't exercise a whole lot," said Elizabeth "Bjay" Woolley.
  (Round-ligament pain refers to pelvic pain when the ligaments are stretched during pregnancy. It's a normal side
  effect of pregnancy.)

- "I was on weightlifting restrictions from early on," said
  Alycia Green. "As the pregnancy progressed, I found it difficult to find the energy to exercise, in addition to the pains
  and discomfort the extra weight caused."

- "I made sure my heart rate [never rose above] 140 beats per
  minute," said Katie, 30, type 1, of Alexandria, Virginia. Her
  daughter is 7 months old. "I quit running at week 12 and did
  the elliptical and bike instead. I was more out of breath than
  usual. I didn't have insulin resistance until I was almost 30
  weeks. I think that's because I was exercising. After [my
  doctors] said the baby was measuring small, they advised
  me to stop exercising altogether, or just take it really slow,
  so I quit."

- "I enjoyed going for walks and playing with my 3-year-old
  daughter until I was not able to any longer," said Christi
  Tipton. "Bed rest and limited activity sound great to a lot of
  people, as people keep telling me, but it is a lot of hard work

to give up control to others, especially with other children. With insulin resistance at an all-time high, [I need] exercise so much more, but with high blood pressure and the need for bed rest, dietary habits are the only way to really control my blood sugar."

- "Because of the high-risk nature of my pregnancy, my ability to exercise was very limited," said Kathryn. "Listen to your body and your doctors."

- "I did a pregnancy yoga DVD almost every day until I was too big and tired to move even that much," said Amy Eddy. "Do what works for you."

No matter how much you're exercising—or not—you're still likely doing everything else you possibly can to stay healthy for yourself and for your future child. That's absolutely the key thing. Remember that perspective is everything. "I think that the most important lesson I learned is that no one is a 'perfect diabetic,'" said Abby Nagel. "You just have it in your mind, body, and soul to remain diligent about testing your blood, eating as healthfully as you can, and making sure your life partner, husband, friends, co-workers know what to do in case of a bad low. While all the testing is time consuming and stressful and seems never ending, the goal is to make sure that you have a healthy baby. The final result is well worth all the things you go through!"

And while it's easy to say when you aren't yet sleep deprived and trying to feed, clothe, and soothe a newborn 'round the clock, try to maintain these great habits down the road. "When I was pregnant, I was the healthiest I had ever been in my life and the sugars were the best ever," said Amy Eddy. "Since having my child, I haven't been so diligent in taking care of myself, three years later! My advice for everyone, including myself, is to take care of *you*. Don't forget *you*. Your baby needs a healthy mommy who's going to be around a while, so don't forget about the things you need to do to ensure that happens."

6

Approaching the Big Day

Your due date is just ahead, and you keep hearing about something called a birth plan. How much can you really plan? Well, there are a number of things to think about. With the vaginal or cesarean delivery option, consider your health history and how things have gone during this pregnancy. What does your doctor suggest and, more important, why? If you're in good control and don't have any health issues, an uncomplicated vaginal birth is definitely possible. Early induction or cesarean birth is common in pregnancies with diabetes, though, and it's good to know why if this is recommended for you. Pre-existing diabetic eye or kidney problems may dictate the kind of birth your health care provider suggests. Amid all the excitement, will you want to work with a doula? What questions should you ask before you hire one, and what questions and advice will she have for you as a woman with diabetes?

Forty Weeks: You Might Not Get That Far (But Maybe You Will)

Typically, pregnant women with diabetes have been told that it's not safe to remain pregnant past a certain time (usually a week or two shy of 40 weeks). You're considered full term around week 38. Studies show that a small number of late-term pregnancies end in miscarriage, stillbirth, or lethal birth defects, leading one 1986 study to conclude that "timing and mode of delivery is individualized, but the general scheme is to induce labor around the thirty-eighth week of pregnancy."[1]

Many doctors stick with this concept for their pregnant patients with diabetes. It's common for a maternal/fetal medicine specialist or a high-risk obstetrician to follow these guidelines, often inducing labor one to two weeks before your due date or scheduling a caesarean birth at that time. "We explain the risks versus the benefits of these protocols and do our best to help patients realize why these recommendations are made," said Dr. Ian Grable. "These are not recommendations made by our own group of doctors. They are made by multiple bodies of committees, based on huge numbers of data, worldwide and national. They're not just small little studies." (See Resources for study citations.)[2]

Some people are fine with the recommendations; I'm one of them. My son was due in April, and four months earlier my obstetrician and I talked about birthing decisions. Because of my eye issues, my obstetrician had consulted with my ophthalmologist. The eye doc recommended (but did not insist) that I deliver either by a scheduled c-section or vaginally using forceps and possibly a vacuum. The concern was that my eyes might not fare so well if I pushed my son out the traditional way, that the pressure changes might cause more damage to the already leaky blood vessels in the back of my eyes. The idea of using forceps to yank my kid out or using a vacuum to suck him out (with the possibility that if he were a larger baby at birth, he might get stuck behind my pubic bone and suffer shoulder damage) sounded incredibly unpleasant for both me and him. On the other hand, a scheduled c-section didn't faze me at all. (I'd had several prior surgeries, including abdominal, for a bunch of entirely different, nondiabetic health issues and already knew what to expect). My goal was simply to ensure that my son and I were happy, healthy, and alive at the end of the day. Therefore, I didn't think twice about scheduling a c-section, and the fact that I am strongly pro-painkiller made it a comfortable and completely lucid experience overall. I was fully awake at, aware of, and amazed by our son's birth and was able to hold him and see him shortly after the procedure. (Plus, I loved knowing exactly when my son would be born). It *is* surgery, though. While I don't want to say having a c-section was a piece of cake, for me it was the safe, healthy, and preferred way to bring my son into the world.

How Natural Can This Birth Be?

Others feel differently, some quite strongly. Some women are natural birth advocates and work with their doctors to try to give birth without using drugs or (many or any) medical interventions.

"First and foremost, I wanted a healthy baby," said Elizabeth Edelman, 28, type 1, of Cleveland, Ohio. Her daughter is 9 months old. "My husband and I attended Bradley classes because I wanted to do a drug-free birth, if possible. I felt that our bodies are designed to give birth and although there is pain, there is a reason for the pain—a baby is coming out of you! Also, I am not a fan of being drugged up. When I was pregnant, I couldn't find one drop of information about type 1 women who delivered their babies without drugs. I'm happy to say that it can be done."

Edelman, who was diagnosed with type 1 about two years before becoming pregnant, had "very, very tight" control during her pregnancy, she said. "I wore a CGM. I tested my blood sugar at least 14 times a day. I counted every carbohydrate that went into my body. I did prenatal yoga. I worked my butt off!" She also had no kidney, nerve, eye, blood pressure, or other medical problems before or during pregnancy that would complicate her health. Edelman also had all the standard fetal monitoring weekly before she went into labor spontaneously in her thirty-ninth week. "Nothing gave the doctors any reason to induce," she said. One of the obstetricians in her practice was "pushing for an induction," and another told her that "the second they saw something out of the ordinary, they would send me for an induction," but that time never came. "They said they didn't want me going past 40 weeks, though, but I never made it [that far]."

While some women have the good fortune to have the birth experience they planned for and perhaps always dreamed of, sometimes it just isn't possible. Circumstances can change—sometimes rapidly—and sometimes the medical team in charge does things differently than you would like, either because of standards ("It's the way it's always done here") or because of a legitimate health concern, resulting in a birth experience that is different from what you would prefer. Regardless of what happens on the day you give birth, keep in mind that it is by no means a competition over how much pain a mother endures or whether she delivers vaginally or by cesarean section.

That said, wishing for one kind of birth experience to have happened instead of the one that did can occur. "I knew myself and didn't expect [to plan for a natural birth]," said Sharon. "I never thought it would be possible with all of the intervention a diabetic pregnancy has. I never allowed myself to dream of a natural birth, though a water birth did always sound like a great idea."

The most important thing, of course, is the arrival of your child, hopefully healthy and happy. Some women say giving birth is a transcendental experience; others think of it as a means to an end. You can be anywhere between those endpoints on the spectrum. With the potential for serious problems at any time during pregnancy, labor, and delivery (with or without diabetes), the key thing is not to feel guilty about requiring medical assistance, medication, or something else.

Another way to look at it is to consider the difference between a wedding and a marriage. A bride can focus on her wedding day and be really upset that some part of the ceremony didn't go the way she wanted it to. Will that set the tone for the rest of the marriage? In the end, the strength of the relationship is more important than the events of one day, just as your health and your baby's health, and the bond you have as mother and child, will likely become more meaningful as you move farther away from what happened on the day you gave birth.

What's a Birth Plan?

Some women have specific ideas about how they want the experience of giving birth to be. If this describes you, think about what is important to you and talk to your doctor about whether your wishes are possible. If there are blanket hospital policies for all pregnant women with diabetes, find out why and how you might be able to work around them if you feel strongly about something specific.

"I used the Internet to download a free fill-in birth plan and gave a copy of it to my OB and to the hospital staff," said Joy McCarren. "I really wanted to be able to have as close to a natural delivery as possible, and also to manage my own insulin needs throughout labor."

Sharon said she agonized over her birth plan, particularly because she wanted to use her insulin pump rather than an insulin drip during labor. "I typed it up and brought it to my OB's office around week 36 or 37 to have them look it over first and let me know if anything didn't seem reasonable, and then put it in my file in Labor & Delivery," she said. "There were a few very emotional appointments when I was getting the message that I would have to be on an insulin drip and the OB team would be totally in charge of my diabetes care." Her endocrinologist wrote her obstetrician's team a detailed letter and committed to being available at any time, day or night, if Sharon couldn't self-manage her insulin or needed help during labor. "My biggest concern

Ingredients for a Birth Plan

"I think birth plans are fine with the realization that things might not go according to plan," said Carol Levy, MD, CDE, senior medical director of endocrinology for Novo Nordisk and an endocrinologist who saw more than 600 pregnant patients with diabetes at Weill-Cornell Medical Center over an eight-year period. These are some (but not all—there may be other things that you value) issues to consider:

- Whether you'll be induced or will be allowed to go into labor up until a certain week or date
- Your ideas on a scheduled c-section
- Your thoughts on a c-section birth if things aren't progressing vaginally
- Where you stand on getting an episiotomy (an incision into the perineum and vagina to help ease delivery)
- Wearing your pump versus using an intravenous (IV) drip that will administer insulin and/or glucose
- Testing your own blood sugars during labor and delivery
- The use of painkillers, IV fluids, and other medications
- The atmosphere in the room where you deliver (requesting certain music or lighting, for example)
- Immediately breast-feeding after birth
- The use of formula if your baby's blood sugar is low at birth
- The use of a pacifier at birth (some 2009 research showed that babies who use a pacifier in their first few weeks are less likely to breast-feed than infants who never use one)[3]
- Whether you can bond immediately with your baby or hospital policy states that all babies of mothers with diabetes go elsewhere for further observation or treatment
- Who will be in the delivery room
- Who will cut the umbilical cord
- Cord blood collection for private or public banking (see below for more details)

was knowing that the ranges for my blood sugar that I'd been using all along, and which were advised by my perinatologist and endo, were not the same as the ones [the obstetrician's team] would use during the hours of labor and delivery."

Sharon worried that her blood sugars might go higher than she wanted during labor, which could have caused her baby's blood sugar to be too low at birth. (At this point, the baby is producing its own insulin and will secrete more to lower its own high blood sugar, transmitted from its mom. This is why newborns of mothers with diabetes are more likely to have low blood sugars at birth.) "I finally came to a place where I hoped to use my pump, but was okay going on an insulin drip as long as I'd be monitored every hour [versus every two-plus hours, which was standard protocol], and I'd be allowed to go as low as 65 mg/dL without treating as a low and would be corrected with a bolus of insulin if I rose above 120," she said.

Things proceeded well, according to Sharon's wishes, and she and her husband ended up testing her blood sugar every 30 to 45 minutes on their own. "The nurses were pretty blown away by how attentive we were to my sugars and commented more than once that clearly, I was the best person to be in charge and that they'd never have been able to control my sugars as well as we were. After all the struggles getting to that place, it was a nice compliment and reassurance that I did know what was best for me and my baby," she said.

A birth plan is exactly that—a plan—and many things can happen that call for it to be modified or changed altogether. For this reason, some people don't even write one. "No, I didn't have a birth plan," said Bethany Rose. "I knew that there were so many unknowns, and I didn't want to create a plan that, in all likelihood, I wouldn't be able to stick to anyway."

Some people are deeply disappointed when their birth plans aren't followed or aren't given any consideration. "I did have a birth plan—I wanted as natural of a delivery as possible," said Allison Herschede. "I did not want an epidural or an episiotomy. I most definitely did not want a c-section." Her first child was in a breech position (meaning the feet or butt are positioned closest to the vaginal opening rather than, as is usual, the head); this is a standard reason to deliver by cesarean if the baby won't turn.[4] "My doctor would not try an external version [a way to try to turn the baby without surgery], so I had to have a cesarean section," she said. "I was not allowed to have a VBAC [vaginal birth after cesarean] with my second because of my diabetes. My doctor said if I had just been gestational, he would have let me. I think that is utter codswallop. Gestational diabetics tend to have bigger babies than type 1s—my babies were seven pounds and eight pounds, respectively."

Sometimes, even if a birth plan isn't followed, things still turn out okay at the end of the day, noted Sara Bancroft. Her son is 1. "I had a birth plan," she said. "The most important points in the plan were to promote bonding and breast-feeding (I specifically requested no pacifiers!) and to be offered pain relief but to try for as natural a birth as possible. I requested to be allowed to carry my pregnancy as long as possible without an induction, as well. I also insisted that I handle my own insulin pump, and if I was unable to do so, my husband would take charge, *not* the nurses."

Things didn't go as she had intended.

No, the doctors had their own plans for my son's birth, and they denied my request to be allowed to go into labor naturally. They did an amniocentesis at 37 weeks to check for lung maturity, and I was induced as soon as the results came back positive. My induction failed after three days in and out of labor, and I was taken for a c-section. Yet another hospital policy was that all infants born to diabetic mothers were taken swiftly to the NICU [Neonatal Intensive Care Unit] for evaluation (where he was immediately given a pacifier, despite my requests)—so much for my plans to bond with my baby and breast-feed immediately.

I wanted as natural a birth as possible, and my birth suite had a whirlpool tub in the bathroom, so I wanted to labor in the water as much as possible. They would not let me in the tub at all because of the monitors I had to be hooked up to for the induction. I also wanted to avoid pain medication, which I did until the c-section. I really wanted to have the baby laid on my chest after birth to breast-feed, but the hospital did not allow that.

I was 37.5 weeks pregnant when my son arrived. I will always believe that if I had not been induced so early (due to the hospital's [blanket] "policy" [for] all diabetic patients [to be treated the same way] despite [the patient's] level of glucose control and health) I could have had a natural birth.

All's well that ends well. It was not the ideal birth situation, but my son and I are healthy and that is all that matters. I have definitely changed many things (including my team of doctors) in hopes that a subsequent pregnancy can have an even better outcome than my first.

What's What: A Primer on Labor and Delivery Terms

Just so you know what everything means when it's time for your child to arrive, here's a quick explanation of words and phrases that you might hear on or before your baby's birth day.

Full Term

A baby is considered full term anytime after week 37 and up to week 42. Babies who arrive sooner are considered preterm and are more likely to have health issues, which can vary depending on how much earlier the infants are born. Because women with diabetes may suffer placental breakdown, it's common either to be induced or to be scheduled for a cesarean section around week 38 or 39. If your doctor is concerned about your baby's lung development (the lungs are among the last body parts to form fully), you may have an amniocentesis to check lung maturity, along with fetal monitoring to see what's up with other elements of your baby's growth.

Induction/Being Induced

Induction is the use of medication to help you go into labor if you haven't begun to do so on your own. You typically go into the hospital the night before the procedure and are examined to determine where your baby's head is located and whether your cervix is effaced, or dilated. If you aren't dilated, a vaginal suppository medication can help artificially soften the cervix. Typically, fetal monitoring takes place throughout the induction, and after six hours a second dose of the drug is administered. At that point, you'll likely be given another drug called Pitocin, which helps stimulate or enhance contractions.

Labor With Vaginal Delivery

If you go into labor on your own, it typically feels like a series of lower-pelvic, menstrual-like cramps. These cramps can come and go every 10 to 15 minutes; check with your doctor about when to call if you have been given the go-ahead to go into labor on your own. Typically, you can stay at home and monitor the pains, which are early uterine contractions, for about two hours, said Mary Beth Bahren, a senior clinical nurse at the Beth Israel Deaconess Medical Center. "With patients with diabetes, the issues of eating get more intense. We often give advice to keep your insulin pump on and to eat lightly. If you are vomiting or there's something wrong, we tell people to come in right away," she said.

It's also uncommon for most pregnant women at or before term to break their water, which typically happens when the force of a contraction ruptures the sac of amniotic fluid. Instead, this usually happens in the hospital, and if necessary a doctor can manually break your water. "This doesn't hurt, and by then, women usually already have an epidural or labor is already going on and you don't care how it will feel," said Bahren.

When you arrive at the hospital in labor, your blood pressure is assessed, you're given a vaginal exam, and fetal/contraction monitoring begins. You're often observed for a couple of hours in labor and delivery, and at this time your cervix begins to soften, changing from a long, closed space to a shorter, open one. (This is effacement.) When you're making progress, which means your cervix is dilated to 10 inches, you're admitted to a labor room. Once the cervix is fully dilated, you're given the go-ahead to start pushing in tandem with the uterine contractions, which are occurring every two to three minutes by labor's end. This entire process can take many hours, and according to how well you and your baby are tolerating the pushing and on where your baby's head is located as it moves through your pelvis, you're encouraged to continue pushing until the baby is out. "Fourteen to fifteen hours is a typical first-time labor, as long as there are no complications," said Bahren. "It's unlikely that someone would labor for 10 minutes for a first-time baby, but Mazel Tov [congratulations] if they do!"

In a pregnancy with diabetes, with the potential for a larger-than-average child, the pushing part is judged a little more closely, said

Bahren. "If there's no progress after two hours, depending on where the baby's head is stationed, a vacuum, forceps, and/or an emergency c-section might be recommended."

Cesarean/C-Section Delivery

With a cesarean section, your baby is delivered through an incision (usually horizontal, just above your bikini line, or vertical if you've had prior ab surgery with this kind of cut). Recovery time is usually longer than from a vaginal birth (a few weeks versus a few days). A planned c-section is scheduled in advance; an emergency c-section is one performed when there is a problem causing fetal distress or you aren't progressing properly after trying to have a vaginal birth. With an emergency c-section, you're moved from a labor room to an operating room and given more medication, a catheter is inserted into your bladder, and things move much more quickly than with a scheduled procedure, which is like a typical operation. A scheduled c-section can take about 50 minutes from beginning to end, while doctors usually want to get into the uterus within 2 minutes after the decision is made to perform an emergency cesarean.

Spinal and Epidural Anesthesia

Spinal and epidural are two of the most common kinds of anesthesia, or pain relief, used during a cesarean section or vaginal delivery. To explain the difference between a spinal and an epidural, think of your body as if it were a tree trunk. When a tree is cut down, the trunk shows rings around its center. Your spinal cord is the center. The first ring around the cord (center) is a sac of fluid, while the next ring around is an open area called the epidural space. With a spinal, medications "like Novocaine-plus," are injected into that first ring, which is the fluid surrounding the cord. With an epidural, the numbing medication is injected into the space, or the the second ring, around the cord. Both procedures are done through an injection into your lower back; a spinal uses a long needle, while an epidural uses a catheter similar to an insulin pump infusion set.

For a scheduled c-section, typically a spinal is used, and this is a one-time injection that lasts about 45 minutes. While the drug is working, you are awake but cannot feel anything below your waist.

When an epidural is given, the catheter is left in the body, so more medication can be administered, if necessary, for a longer labor. Some people don't like the idea of an epidural, said Bahren, because it can slow labor down and prevents you from being able to leave your bed or walk around during labor. It also doesn't let gravity work to nudge the baby's head downward through the birth canal.

If you do have an epidural and can't feel the force of your contractions, you might be given Pitocin to help you sharpen the feeling so you know when to push. Talk to your doctor if you have any questions or concerns about these forms of anesthesia or medications.

Episiotomy

An episiotomy is a procedure in which an incision is made in the perineum and the vaginal opening that creates more space for the baby to come through. The idea is that creating this space can help prevent the vagina from tearing, said Bahren, although it is possible to have tears even with an episiotomy. Again, talk to your doctor about the pros and cons of an episiotomy and whether it could be used in your case.

Forceps or Vacuum Extraction

Forceps and a vacuum extractor are tools (tongs and a suction cup device, respectively) used to pull the baby out of the birth canal if it gets stuck or otherwise isn't progressing despite much effort on the mom's part—or, as I was advised, if medical considerations prevent you from pushing during labor. These tools are safe for both mom and baby, though only a small number of births actually end up requiring their use. If you still can't deliver the baby vaginally after using these methods, you may need to have a cesarean delivery.

How Diabetes Complications Can Affect the Kind of Birth You Have

Some people don't have pre-existing diabetes or other complications and don't have any health issues during pregnancy. For those of us with diabetes, something about the condition may dictate that one particular thing be done rather than another. I've already mentioned my scheduled c-section because of retinopathy; there are other scenarios, too.

"I had a planned c-section at 36 weeks and 1 day and diabetes played a huge role in that," said Bethany Rose. "The initial plan had been to induce me at (or slightly before) 38 weeks. Around 30 weeks, I started to have problems with my blood pressure going up very quickly. Even quitting work and starting on medication didn't keep it from rising. By the time I had the c-section, I officially had pre-eclampsia." She went for an amnio at 36 weeks on a Friday, and her daughter's lungs weren't fully developed. Rose's doctor scheduled a c-section for the following Monday. On Saturday around noon, Rose's retinopathy caused a hemorrhage in her left eye. "It was one of the scariest things I'd ever experienced—it was horrible," she said. "I contacted my OB, he made some quick arrangements, and by Saturday evening, my baby was born via c-section."

While complications do occur, sometimes it's more the fear of possible problems that make things go the way they do.

"I knew that, more than likely, I would have to be hooked up to an IV, as that is standard practice at my hospital for diabetics, but I hoped to avoid all drugs and not have to use the IV if at all possible," said Joy McCarren. "I had to be induced, which I'd hoped to avoid. The induction did not work, however, and I ended up having a c-section. If I'd not been induced, the doctors had told me that they would prep me for an IV to be inserted, but that unless absolutely necessary, I wouldn't have to be hooked up. This would have left me free to move around on my own and change positions, etc., as often and as much as I'd wanted." McCarren was 40 weeks and 2 days when her daughter was born and had fought with her doctors to go to 40 weeks without interventions. "They had wanted to induce me at 38 weeks, which is standard practice for diabetics," she said. "Because I had kept tight control throughout my pregnancy and because the baby was not measuring large and there were no other complications, I was allowed to go to 40 weeks. That fell on a Sunday, so they tried to induce me on Monday. When that was unsuccessful, they did a c-section on Tuesday, two days after my due date."

Overall, she said, the experience "wasn't bad, but I know if I hadn't been diabetic, I probably wouldn't have had to be induced or have a c-section. I feel things turned out the way they should have, and in the end, was happy with how things went—probably because I had my baby. If I ever want to attempt to have a vaginal delivery, I will have to go to a different hospital, so that is something to consider. I would be willing to have another c-section, even though the recovery time is longer, to be able to deliver closer to home."

Alycia Green had wanted to deliver vaginally and then immediately bond with and breast-feed her son. "I had a birth plan, but I found that everything I had read about birth plans 'going out the window' when the time came was accurate," she said. "My son was breech for most of the pregnancy, so I had to have a c-section instead of a vaginal birth. His blood sugars were low [at birth], so I was not able to see him immediately. The NICU took him and tried to get blood sugars up by dipping a pacifier into a glucose solution and also by feeding him formula—something I honestly did not want. Those measures were insufficient, so they had to put him on an IV. I felt so horrible. I had excellent control throughout the pregnancy and did not anticipate any big problems. I felt so guilty."

It's hard to keep in mind in the heat of the moment, or even in the hazy, sleep-deprived time after giving birth, but often things just happen. Don't beat yourself up if your child is premature or has other health problems. Grieve for what you have to grieve for, but focus on what comes next and what you (and the hospital and the doctors) will do to help get your baby the care required to thrive and be healthy.

What and When To Pack

Filling a bag before you have to leave for the hospital is a great idea; you don't want to be caught unaware if your water breaks unexpectedly and you need to get out the door. (Tip: Put a waterproof sheet under your bedding in your eighth month, suggests Abby Nagel. "If your water breaks, it will not ruin your mattress. We put on the sheet the night before my water broke and the sheets were salvageable—just needed to be put in the washing machine.") You can decide when to pack (some women go into labor weeks before their due dates), but here are some suggestions on what to bring:

Clothing for You

I wore the hospital johnnies (gowns) because they were comfortable and I didn't have to worry about staining them. Not to be too graphic, but a lot of stuff is still coming out of you after giving birth, even if you had a c-section. "Leave at home your own pajamas," said Elizabeth Edelman. "I brought mine and not only were they way too small (pre-pregnancy size, what was I thinking?), but you're leaking blood and all sorts of stuff afterward and you don't want to ruin your clothes!" Other women find their own pajamas or robe comforting and preferable to the hospital johnnies, which always seem to require an advanced degree to cover your entire body properly. (Hint: wear one backward and another on top of it forward. Instant coverage.)

Of course, once the baby's here, no one is (or should be) checking you out for your sense of style. Also, though the baby is now out of you, you will not suddenly become fashion-model slim. Leave your skinny jeans at home and think comfort. "I had brought a lot of my own loose-fitting clothes to wear after the c-section, but I really didn't feel like wearing anything around my waist until about the fourth day, so I stayed in the hospital gown for most of my stay," said Bethany Rose.

The hospital will likely give you giant maxi-pads to handle the flow (officially known as lochia, which can last up to six weeks postpartum and contains blood and bits of your uterine lining) and may have mesh underwear that you can wear in addition to the pads. These disposable undies mean you won't have to soak any intimates in Woolite to take out stains—just chuck 'em and put on a new pair. If you prefer to wear your own, though, bigger might be better: "Make sure to bring some granny panties if you have a c-section; bikinis will cut into your incision," said Allison Herschede. And while many hospitals offer warm socks with traction grips on the soles, others do not, so pack comfortable socks or footwear. "What was super essential to me were footie socks, because those hospital floors get cold and dirty," said Alycia Green. If you plan to breast-feed, you may already have a nursing bra (a bra with cups that open in front for the baby to nurse easily) or other breast-feeding things such as pads or a nursing pillow, but ask your obstetrician ahead of time if you'll be able to get fitted for and buy nursing bras, tank tops, and other nursing items while you are ensconced on the maternity floor. "I had my nursing bra and loose pajamas that opened in the front for easy nursing, but nothing I'd care about if it got soiled," said Sharon. Depending on whether you have an uneventful vaginal delivery or a cesarean, you might be in the hospital anywhere from 24 hours to a few days, so pack accordingly. And finally, for the trip home, bring comfortable clothes that won't bind, chafe, or be ruined if you leak breast milk or get spit up, peed, or pooped on.

Diabetes Gear for You

When it comes to whatever you need to manage your diabetes during and after giving birth, presume that nothing will be available in the hospital. It's better to take everything you need than to be caught empty-handed. "Bring all your diabetes supplies in advance," said Dr. Carol Levy.

This includes all pump and CGM supplies if you use them, extra batteries for your pump, CGM, or meter, insulin syringes if you're on multiple daily injections, alcohol swabs and any other wipes you use, your own meter, glucose test strips, finger-pricker and extra lancets, snacks and glucose sources to treat insulin reactions, and an extra bottle of insulin, even though you're in a hospital and insulin should be readily available. (Again, never presume anything). "Most hospitals don't have pump supplies available," said Dr. Levy. "Plan for the worst and have everything available to you." A good rule, which I followed, is to pack twice as many supplies as you think you will need for the time you are away from home (you never know when something might malfunction). "I brought a list of my insulin ratios, current and pre-pregnancy," said Joy McCarren. While this is good info to have handy, your endocrinologist should be able to tell you what your insulin needs will be postpartum. Also, bring any other drugs you took during pregnancy and might continue, such as thyroid meds, and let your doctor know what they are. Hospital policy might require that you take only the hospital's medications, but it's good to have your own stuff on hand just in case.

"I brought lots of snacks so I wouldn't have to constantly be asking the nurses when I needed a blood sugar boost," said Bethany Rose. Michelle Kowalski took a similar tack: "I made sure I brought some fast-acting sugar with me in case I went low. It turned out to be a good idea as I found myself in the 60s at one point." As mentioned, insulin needs drop dramatically after giving birth, and breast-feeding can cause lows as well, so it is essential to have something within reach for treating hypoglycemic episodes.

Toiletries for You

Although you're staying in a hospital and not a hotel, a nurse may be able to bring you something you have left at home, such as toothpaste or shampoo. But if you want to use all your own personal items, consider the following list: toothbrush, toothpaste, deodorant, shampoo, conditioner, soap, comb or brush, cosmetics, accessories to pull your hair off your face, and anything else you use daily. The hospital will probably have maxi-pads, as well as ice packs and other things to help you feel better after giving birth. Then again, you may prefer to use your own. "I recommend bringing your own pads, as the ones the hospital provides are huge and uncomfortable," said Allison Herschede. "Just don't take anything with you that you don't really need or that isn't essential for your comfort," said Amy Eddy.

Clothes, Gear, and Toiletries for Your Partner

If your partner (and by partner I mean your spouse, boyfriend, girl-friend, or anyone else who's giving you support while you have this baby; if future references to this person are male and you have a female partner, please sub in the correct pronoun) plans to stay in the hospital with you, he should pack what he'd typically pack for an overnight or few days' stay away from home. In particular, make sure he packs sweatpants or pajamas for the overnights. The only tushies the nurses and hospital staff want to see are tiny newborn ones—not your partner's when he's sprawled fast asleep in skimpy tighty whities across the easy chair pushed into the corner in your hospital room.

Entertainment might come in handy if your labor is particularly long. "My husband and I watched movies and listened to music on the laptop while I was laboring through the induction," said Sara Bancroft. "It was such a great idea for my husband to bring it." Speaking of entertainment, it can be a good idea to have something to do if you find yourself (as my husband and I did) waiting a while before going in for a scheduled c-section; I read through a few magazines while my husband, who prides himself on being a handy fellow, took it upon himself to "fix" a piece of monitoring equipment that a nurse couldn't figure out how to work. The woman thought the machine was plugged in properly, but Dave—my Registered Professional Electrical Engineer husband—noticed that she had examined the wrong cord. "Once I saw her fooling with a data cord and not a power cord, I knew I had to take over," he said. "As soon as she left, I checked and found the power cord had come out from the back of the piece of equipment, so I plugged that back in. Voilà! The machine worked!" (Dave asked me to make sure he came across as "brilliant" in this particular anecdote, so here you go. His website is www.duncanengineering.com and he is free for consulting projects.)

Other people may be more content to surf their BlackBerries, read, write in a journal, or do other things, and some people—particularly those in quick, active labor—never even touch the stuff. "I took books, music, and handheld games, but found I really didn't use them," said Joy McCarren. "If your labor is long, you may want those things, but really you are pretty distracted so don't need all that stuff. Plus, once baby comes, you have no time for those things at the hospital. Your partner may want a book or magazine, though, because he will be sitting around awake a lot more than you will be." He may also want to bring his own snacks and drinks, particularly if your hospital room has its own fridge.

Stuff for Baby

Your baby comes into the world with nothing but leaves the hospital with more items than you ever thought a small being could need. Luckily, many of these things will be provided by the hospital. What you need to bring is a going-home outfit, including socks and a hat, and a fully installed car seat (check what the car seat policy is if you live in a city and plan to take a taxi home from the hospital). Depending on the weather and the time of year, a blanket for warmth in the car seat might be a good idea. Just about everything else—a stack of diapers, bathing items such as a nasal aspirator, formula if you started using it, feeding items such as a tube for finger feeding if breast-feeding didn't go well from the start, and any other items that are being used from an open container (such as a partially started container of formula or a pack of diapers)—is yours to keep. Just make sure you have enough space for whatever you end up lugging back home. "I highly advise bringing a suitcase with plenty of room, because there is so much stuff to bring home," said Anna Tang Norton.

Anything Else

If there's something that will make you feel much more comfortable, such as a favorite pillow or quilt, feel free to bring it—though the hospital will certainly have enough standard ones to go around. A notepad and pen can come in handy if you are taking notes about anything—blood sugars, changing insulin ratios, insight about becoming a parent, or whatever. Definitely bring a list of people to call and e-mail once your baby has arrived, along with your cell phone, the phone charger, and even your laptop (or lots of change for a public pay phone). If you plan to film or photograph anything, remember your camera, videocamera, extra batteries or the charger, and film (for a nondigital camera). For some, the choice of music is important; consider whether you want a loaded-up laptop, mp3 player, CD player, or something else to play your favorite tunes.

Don't forget other things that you probably already have tucked away in your purse or wallet, such as your health insurance card, copies of your birth plan if you have one, and your endocrinologist's and other doctors' phone numbers.

Working With a Doula

A doula can provide nonmedical assistance before, during, and after giving birth—and that care can be emotional, physical, informational, or practical. "A doula is really there to support the mom the way we would have done 100 years ago—with women supporting women in labor," said Stefanie Antunes, LCCE, CD (DONA), CHBE, director of public relations for DONA International, the world's largest and oldest doula association. "A doula can provide things to help with labor progression, suggest position changes and other things the mom can do. Postpartum, a doula can help with breast-feeding and make sure the mom has all the help she needs. A doula can also help with the transition to parenthood and how a couple will adjust to life with a new baby, help with siblings, and light housekeeping," she said. Birthing doulas can offer help through a few sessions before you give birth and support on the day itself, and they may come back for appointments after the birth to answer any questions and to help with breast-feeding issues; postpartum doulas are strictly for assistance after the baby arrives.

Doulas can help reduce the number of interventions during delivery, and women who work with doulas are less likely to have cesarean births or deal with postpartum depression, said Antunes. "Most of the time, a woman with pre-existing diabetes is not going to go into labor on her own. A doula can show research and studies to show the pros and cons [of different interventions] so that the mom can be comfortable making a decision. Maybe there's another option that might be better suited" to that woman and her specific health history, she said.

A doula can be useful before and during a cesarean delivery, too. Because a woman isn't laboring or pushing during a c-section birth, her body may not get the physical cues it would get during a vaginal birth that a baby will soon be ready to nurse. Before the delivery, a doula can help a new mom-to-be figure out how to use a breast pump to collect colostrum (liquid particularly high in antibodies and minerals that is produced in the breasts just before and after giving birth) to feed the baby at birth if the infant's blood sugar is low, rather than feeding the baby formula, which some mothers prefer to avoid. "Skin-to-skin contact in the first hour can also elevate a baby's blood sugar level, and it can really help avoid needing to supplement," said Antunes. "The odds of having a baby with hypoglycemia are higher in mothers with diabetes, and this may undermine the breast-feeding process getting started," she said. A doula can focus entirely on the new mom's needs. "A doula is really for helping a woman focus on the transition to new motherhood, versus a health provider's role, which is to make sure the mom and baby are safe," said Antunes.

"I found a doula who was from my hometown who was also a type 1 diabetic—that sealed the deal," said Bethany Rose. Rose wanted to work with a doula because she "felt like I had no clue about how to have a baby and I wanted to make the process go as smoothly as possible. I knew, as a high-risk pregnancy because of the diabetes, that I would be working with an OB/GYN, and figured that a midwife wasn't quite what I was looking for as a result. I didn't need the medical side of things from this person, just the experience and support." Rose's doula had prepared to be with the parents-to-be during labor and delivery; when Rose ended up needing an emergency c-section, her doula was not allowed in the room during the procedure but offered support and made sure Rose got answers to her questions before the surgery. "She then did the same after the c-section. I was shaking quite badly afterwards and she did some massage to help me feel better, and offered a lot of encouragement," said Rose.

Other women who worked with doulas say they wanted an objective and knowledgeable person with them during labor, in addition to a relative. "Having an experienced non–family member woman there to support the birthing mother is invaluable, not only to help the laboring woman manage the physical and emotional ups and downs of labor and delivery, but to provide a calming and reassuring presence for any other family member who might be present," said Clemma Muller. "Also, having the doula as a consistent presence throughout a long labor, when nursing shifts might change two, three, or even more times, is very nice."

A doula can guide you through a birth experience with unexpected health issues. Betsy Fuller Matambanadzo, 34, type 1, of Brooklyn, New York, wanted a natural birth but sought a doula around week 34 when she felt her doctor was strongly suggesting induction at week 37 because of the baby's size. "Because of my apprehension and worry that I would not be able to properly determine which interventions were necessary, I hired a doula," she said. She was about to have an amnio to determine whether the baby's lungs were developed enough but chose to induce when she learned at 37 weeks that she had obstetric cholestasis (a temporary liver condition—unrelated to diabetes—that has a higher risk of causing stillbirth late in pregnancy). The induction did not work: Matambanadzo labored for four days, with increasing amounts of Pitocin, but her cervix never fully dilated. A doctor broke her water, but instead of delivering, Matambanadzo developed a uterine infection. She ultimately chose to have an epidural and a c-section, and her son is now 3.

"My doula was incredible," said Matambanadzo. "She was by my side when my husband needed to get away, and helped me ask the right questions about every intervention medical staff suggested or performed, and advocated for minimized cervical checks [a manual exam to check whether the cervix is dilated], which had felt invasive and uncomfortable for me."

Finding a doula with whom you mesh well is important; it's probably best to hire someone who shares your philosophies of, say, pain control during labor or breast-feeding. "In theory, a doula is supposed to be truly objective, but I could see how it might be difficult to be truly objective when it comes to something this big and important and emotional," said Bethany Rose.

Doulas typically cost between $600 and $1,000, with those in rural areas charging less and those in cities charging up to $1,500, said DONA's Antunes. In October 2009, doulas became a classification for third-party insurance codes, which means a U.S. health insurance company may be more likely to cover some or all of the cost of hiring a doula. Doulas have been covered in the past under Medicaid and as a one-off expense through some U.S. insurance companies, said Antunes.

How to Find and What to Ask a Potential Doula

While DONA International certifies doulas and its members (who are both certified and uncertified) and follows a code of ethics, the doula industry is unregulated. Anyone can call herself a doula. The association has a database where you can find doulas based near where you are located and offers the following questions as a starting point for finding the right doula:[5]

For Any Doula

- What training have you had? (If a doula is certified, you might consider checking with the organization.)

- Do you have one or more backup doulas for times when you are not available? May we meet her or them?

- What is your fee, what does it include, and what are your refund policies?

When Interviewing a Birth Doula

- Tell me about your experience as a birth doula.

- What is your philosophy about birth and supporting women and their partners through labor?

- May we meet to discuss our birth plans and the role you will play in supporting me through birth?

- May we call you with questions or concerns before and after the birth?

- When do you try to join women in labor? Do you come to our home or meet us at the place of birth?

- Do you meet with us after the birth to review the labor and answer questions?

When Interviewing a Postpartum Doula

- Tell me about your experience as a postpartum doula.

- What is your philosophy about parenting and supporting women and their families postpartum?

- May we meet to discuss our postpartum needs and the role you will play in supporting us in the postpartum period?

- May we call you with postpartum questions or concerns before the birth?

- When do your services begin after birth?

- What is your experience in breast-feeding support?

- Have you had a criminal background check and a recent TB test, and do you have current CPR certification?

Source: DONA International.

If you hire a doula, talk to her specifically about what to bring on the day you give birth. "Check with your doula to see if they are planning on bringing anything as well," said Yehudit W. "We purchased a birthing ball/yoga kit for the birth, which was a bit on the expensive side, but when our doula showed up with one in tow, we ended up returning ours to the store."

Also, let your obstetrician know that you are working with a doula. While it is your right to hire whomever you want, and while many doctors will be fine with a doula in the room, others may not. In late 2009, a clinic in Utah posted a sign at its entrance explaining that it would no longer work with women who wanted to hire doulas, use a birth plan, or deliver using the Bradley natural childbirth philosophy. "For those patients who are interested in such methods, please notify the nurse so we may arrange transfer of your care," the sign reads.[6]

Cord Blood Banking

Cord blood banking is an option for all new parents to consider. Cord blood, collected from the newborn's umbilical cord and the placenta after the cord has been clamped, contains adult stem cells that can be developed into many of the different cells of the body. Neither mom nor baby feels any pain when cord blood is collected. Storing this blood, in either a public or a private cord blood bank, means that the stem cells can be used in the future.

Why would you want or need to collect and store cord blood? Currently, cord blood is being used to help treat some forms of leukemia, lymphoma, and other rarer diseases, and research is ongoing to see how cord blood might help people with other conditions, including type 1 diabetes. However, knowledge in this area is still evolving, and currently there's no guarantee that cord blood will help a child recently diagnosed with type 1 or type 2 diabetes. And, for some conditions, it's possible that the stored cord blood contains the same genetic abnormalities that caused the condition in the first place.

Michael J. Haller, MD, an assistant professor at the University of Florida in Gainesville, is exploring whether cord blood stem cells have the potential to slow the process that breaks down insulin-producing cells in kids with newly diagnosed type 1 diabetes. "While this research is in its earliest stages, there is undoubtedly great promise in the potential for cord blood–based therapies to one day make a tangible difference in the treatment and perhaps prevention of type 1 diabetes," he said.[7]

Practical applications of cord blood to treat diabetes are a long way off. In the meantime, parents can consider collecting cord blood and storing it at a private cord blood bank or donating it to a public cord blood bank.

What's the difference?

A private bank will pick up the blood from the hospital when your baby is born and store it in its own facility. There is an upfront charge of $1,500 to $2,000 for this service, and annual storage fees are several hundred dollars. In the event that you want to use the blood, it will be available to you directly.

A public bank collectively stores blood and does not charge a fee to parents who donate there. The blood can be used by anyone who needs it, and should you want to retrieve the blood you stored, it's highly unlikely you will get your exact donation in return. You give up ownership to your donation once you decide to bank publicly.

If you choose not to bank your newborn's cord blood, it is discarded as medical waste.

Should you consider collecting your child's cord blood? The cost of private banking isn't insignificant for many parents, but it's the only way to retain ownership of those stem cells. Public banking is a growing choice (currently, Dr. Haller estimates that only 5 percent of all available cord blood is banked this way), and like a conventional blood bank, the public bank makes stem cells available if there's a need for them.

As mentioned, if your child develops a disease where cord blood could be beneficial, the child's own cord blood may contain the same genetic mutations that caused the disease. In this case, the child's cord blood will not be useful. However, if a child's sibling has the illness that cord blood could help, that sibling's cord blood is more likely to be a genetic match.

"Whether or not to store cord blood for your newborn is a difficult decision for almost any parent," said Dr. Haller. "The decision is even more difficult when a parent knows their child may be at increased risk for developing a disease that someday might be treated or at least helped with the use of the cells collected at birth. Parents must weigh the potential theoretical benefits of having cord blood stored (as there are currently no established therapies using these cells) with the risks (i.e., cost) of storage. In the end, there is no right or wrong answer, but parents should make an informed decision after reviewing their options. If parents decide not to privately bank the cord blood, they should at the very least make an effort to donate the cord blood to a public bank in order to support the greater good of society and potentially provide a lifesaving therapy to someone suffering from a malignancy." (He noted that if just a small additional fraction of cord blood from U.S. births were publicly stored, the need for bone marrow donor banks would essentially be eliminated.)

If you decide to bank your child's cord blood, talk to your obstetrician about collection (your obstetrician is the one who collects it) and whether there is a small fee for doing so (many doctors do this for free, but you never know). You need to decide by a certain date—week 30 of your pregnancy or so—and whether you choose to work with a private or public bank, you need to fill out paperwork and make sure everything is in order well before you give birth.

If you feel that private cord blood banking isn't feasible for financial or other reasons, don't beat yourself up about it. "Given that there are still no established therapies for cord blood in treating diabetes (outside of research protocols), families should not feel guilty or as if they have wronged their child if they are unable to or decide not to store the cord blood privately," said Dr. Haller.

You're So Close

At this point, the finish line seems just ahead. It may feel like you've been pregnant forever, but the end really is near. Try to relish the final few weeks of pregnancy, despite wherever your blood sugars land every moment, whatever you're eating these days, and however you are handling the heft and aches that typify the end of the third trimester of pregnancy. And on the day you have your baby, try to take everything in—not just what your blood sugars are doing.

"You're giving birth to a baby and you are not just a person with diabetes," said Dr. Carol Levy. On the day they deliver, "typically, people with diabetes want to control everything, but there are other doctors there who will be able to handle things, usually. Don't forget to bring your list of people to call. Try to enjoy it."

Hello, Mama!

7

The Big Day

It's here! There's a lot going on today, and your diabetes care is just one part of the bigger picture. But it's an important one, and knowing the answers to certain questions will make the day go more smoothly:

- Will you be allowed to check your own blood sugars while preparing for labor, or will someone else be in charge?
- Should you keep your pump on and manage your own needs or use an insulin drip and have a medical person oversee the dosage?
- What will you do if you have a low blood sugar but aren't supposed to eat anything?
- What will happen if you need an emergency cesarean?
- What can you expect to happen once your child is born, with or without any complications?
- And who's going to hold your meter in the moments after your baby's arrival?

After all, if this is your first child, it's not just the birthday of your new-born but also the first day of your life as a parent who happens to have diabetes. Welcome, Mama!

Ideally, you read Chapter 6 weeks if not months ago and you've talked to your doctors extensively about what to expect today, with both your diabetes and your delivery. Maybe you took childbirth classes at your hospital and you're as prepared as you can be.

Or maybe not.

"Expect the unexpected," said Joy McCarren. "Even with lots of careful planning, things tend not to go as planned, and often go in a way you never thought they would. It's good to remain flexible and relaxed as much as possible. Just keep in mind that even if you have to deviate from your plan, in the end you will have your baby and that is what it is all about."

Diabetes While Delivering

So who will handle your insulin needs, your blood sugar tests, and the treatment of low or high sugars while you are in labor or having a c-section? Many women say they prefer to handle it themselves; others want someone else to manage the details so that they can focus solely on having a baby. Your hospital's policy may dictate that a team of doctors or nurses will oversee insulin drip administration, blood sugar management, and what can and cannot be eaten to treat a low. See whether you can share some of the responsibilities: you and your partner might get the okay to handle checking your blood sugar on your own meter, for example, while other things such as the insulin drip are managed by the health care team.

Here are some specific details you might want to discuss before you deliver:

Insulin Drip

An insulin drip provides a steady stream of insulin through a catheter inserted into one of your veins. If your blood sugars spike or plummet, the rate of insulin delivery can be adjusted more quickly with a drip than with a pump. Some doctors really like using a drip because of how effective it can be.

"I prefer an insulin drip," said Dr. Carol Levy. "Because of the fluid shifts that can happen during labor, your blood pressure can change. That can impair delivery of insulin via the pump. With glucose shifts and an intravenous drip, we can boost up the insulin rate much faster and can adjust in a much more rapid fashion. It works immediately." Low blood pressure or edema (extra fluid under the skin) can inhibit the absorption of insulin delivered under the skin; with a IV drip, the insulin always gets into the body efficiently.

For a scheduled c-section, Dr. Levy said she has no problem with a patient who wants to keep using her insulin pump. Other doctors, hospital protocols, and safety concerns mandate the use of an insulin drip, especially during an unscheduled cesarean. An insulin drip can be adjusted easily by a health care team, while it's unlikely the same team will be able to adjust your own pump if you cannot do it yourself for some reason.

If you want to wear your pump while you deliver, ask your obstetrician and your endo how they typically handle insulin delivery during the birthing process. You may want to keep your insulin pump on because you're so used to handling changes yourself. For some people, the better choice is obvious: "I was allowed to keep my pump on with my first delivery, and my blood sugars were perfect," said Allison Herschede. "With my second, I was not allowed to wear it and was supposed to be on an insulin drip. The doctor neglected to start the drip even well after the baby was born, for fear that I would go low. The next morning, I was 200 and put my pump back on against medical advice. My numbers were perfect after that."

Before anything gets started in the labor and delivery room, or in the operating room if you're having a c-section, know exactly how you and your endo want your insulin needs to be managed throughout the process. (This chat will most likely occur during one of the last appointments you expect to have with your endo before giving birth.) Double check things with the obstetrics staff at the hospital when you arrive to have your baby; in particular, check with the anesthesiologist. The anesthesiologist often controls which medications are used in an operating room if you know you will have (or think you might have) a cesarean or might otherwise need anesthesia. "Make sure you've spoken with your endocrinologist prior to coming in about what you should tell hospital obstetricians, high-risk OB fellows, and residents, and so on," said Dr. Levy. "They may not know what the plan is, for example, about whether your endocrinologist wants you to stay on your pump, or if you should go on an insulin drip right away." If there's a discrepancy between what your endo prefers and what the obstetrician prefers, it's better to have that conversation in a doctor's office weeks before giving birth than in the hospital while waiting to deliver. Better yet, write down all the details and get your endo to sign the note with her contact information. This can be particularly helpful if you are delivering at a hospital where your endocrinologist does not have privileges to see patients.

Blood Sugar Testing

You'll probably be allowed to test your blood sugar throughout your delivery, though your hospital's protocol may require that you test on in-house meters so there's an official record. (You can bring your own meter and test on that as well.) If you think you might have trouble managing the machinery on your own, teach your partner how to test your sugar (which may include how to operate your meter, how to obtain a drop of blood from a fingerstick, and how to work your insulin pump and/or CGM). There may be times—when you're in active labor, for example, or feeling nauseous during a c-section—when you don't feel comfortable or able to check your own blood sugar. Having a knowledgeable partner can come in handy, as the hospital's medical staff are unlikely to know exactly how your particular meter works or may be unwilling to have anything to do with your own medical devices for legal reasons.

"With my first pregnancy, the hospital had a policy that I could only use their meter," said Abby Nagel, "even though when I used my own meter, the readings were virtually identical. Since my endo did not practice at the hospital I delivered at, I did not have the over-sight I needed to adjust my fluctuating sugars after the birth. That was hard to manage. For my second pregnancy, I had the same issue at a different hospital, but my OB had an endo for me to work with. Unfortunately, [the hospital's endocrinologist] did not listen to me and set up basal rates that were too high. After crashing numerous times, I basically told him to listen to me, or I would hold him responsible for bad treatment. He relented and at my request started working with my own endo to adjust my basal rates daily."

Nagel's takeaway: "Be very vigilant when dealing with these types of issues, and be your own advocate to make sure things are done cor-rectly." Your vigilance can also cover frequency of testing and treat-ing low blood sugars. If your medical team insists on testing you every two hours but they're late, there's no reason you can't test on your own more frequently and on your own meter. Likewise, having your own stash of fast-acting sugar can help you treat a low immediately instead of being forced to wait for a hospital staffer to tend to you.

Infusion Set and CGM Sensor Location

If you're using an insulin pump or a CGM, ensure that the pump's infusion set or the CGM sensor is placed somewhere it won't be disturbed if you need to have an unexpected c-section. Higher on the abdomen or on the hip should be fine, or on any arm or leg site you have used before so that you know how well you absorb insulin from that area. Double check with your obstetrician ahead of time exactly which part of the body you should avoid. Bring extra supplies in case the site stops working and you need to change the location right away.

Insulin Doses and Blood Sugars: What Happens Now?

You've likely been testing and correcting your blood sugars for months if not years (particularly if it took you a while to conceive and you were maintaining tight control before pregnancy), so don't let up just as you're about to cross the finish line. Great numbers during labor and delivery will lower the risk of your baby being born with high blood sugars. Remember: when your sugars go up, your baby's blood sugar does the same, but because the child isn't diabetic inside the uterus, he or she is also producing insulin to bring the high down. This can result in macrosomia (an oversized baby), and it can also cause your infant to have very low blood sugars at birth. After the umbilical cord has been cut, the extra insulin already produced by the baby's body may remain, but the baby's blood sugar is no longer being elevated because yours is; as a result, being born can send the newborn's blood sugar plummeting too far.

The baby will have blood sugar level checks no later than one hour after birth, and then hourly until sugars are stable, said Dr. Tamara Takoudes. "Every hospital has a slightly different cutoff for 'normal,' but the values are lower than those for adults. Above 40 mg/dL is normal for a newborn."

Hypoglycemia at birth can require immediate treatment, usually with formula or a glucose solution and typically by bottle, and this might not be the welcome-to-the-world experience you'd like your child (or you or your partner) to have.

So how often should you test your blood sugar while you're in labor or while you are having a cesarean? A scheduled c-section should last less than an hour if there are no complications; an emergency c-section can be quicker, and vaginal deliveries can take many hours. I tested several times on the morning of my c-section, about once an hour, and probably twice during the procedure itself. Figure out the schedule that works best for you, and keep in mind that the hospital may ask to test your blood sugar on its machines to a particular schedule, such as every two hours. As long as you're aware of what's going on, test as often as you're comfortable with. If you have a CGM, you might avoid this issue for the most part, but do make sure that the device is trending accurately against the numbers your meter gave when you tested earlier in the day.

"What I often tell people is that it's very important to keep blood sugar in tight range during labor and delivery," said Dr. Levy. "If mom has high blood sugars, it may increase the risk of the baby having hypoglycemia. My goal for patients is to be between 70 and 90 mg/dL, but it is not always perfectly achieved." Other doctors and hospitals have higher goals for blood sugars during labor: "Generally less than 120 mg/dL is the goal, and some patients may experience severe hypoglycemia with these lower goals," said Dr. Tamara Takoudes.

What if you're a bit higher than the goal range at some point? Do you need to be concerned about a slight excursion? "We can't give a definitive answer on that," Dr. Carol Levy said. "It's less likely to be a problem if you are 120 mg/dL for 45 minutes, instead of being 400 mg/dL for three hours."

Remember, too, that blood sugars can change immediately after you give birth. For some, they soar; for others, they nose-dive.

"I wore my pump the entire time and never went above 90 until the baby was delivered," said Sharon. "We were concerned about plummeting sugar once the placenta was delivered, so we lowered my basal at that point. I also had a 50 percent dextrose drip started, which turned out to be overkill. I rose quickly to about 270 while still in surgery, but my husband was able to bolus, and within a few hours, I was back in the normal range."

Joy McCarren found herself at the other end of the spectrum. "My blood sugars were okay until a few hours after delivery, when they started to go down rather quickly," she said. "I wasn't able to eat anything that first day after my c-section, so I was thankful to have my pump to adjust my insulin needs accordingly. By that first night, I started having severe lows, and my insulin needs were dropping back to about what they were pre-pregnancy." Lowering pump basal rates and insulin-to-carb ratios immediately after delivering can help prevent such lows happening—even hours after giving birth.

If you are keeping records of your own blood sugars, food intake, and so on, don't be surprised if the hospital staff doesn't get what you're doing. "I was not at all prepared for the treatment I received in the hospital," said Katie. "I was supposed to be the one who handled my blood sugar control, but the nurses had no idea what their role should be. They were breathing down my neck asking to see my blood glucose log. I keep my log on a website, and I'm not used to writing it on paper. But I wrote it down, in tiny numbers, because there was *not* enough room on the outdated log they gave me. They would come in and study it, and say they wanted to copy it. I was like, 'Okay, sure. Go ahead,' but they never did. I guess they were worried that I might go low or something, but I reassured every nurse that I had dealt with this for 23 years and knew how to manage it. I dreaded every shift change because a new nurse would come in, ask me whether I was testing my blood glucose, what my numbers had been, and what I should be eating. We had tons of visitors, and a lot of them brought carby food; the nurses acted like food police a little bit. I just ignored them; I wasn't hungry anyway because I'd had a c-section, so my husband ate all the food."

If you're using both your own meter and a hospital meter to track your numbers, keep in mind that they may give different readings—as much as 20 percent off. So if you're at 100 mg/dL, one meter might say you're at 80 m/dL and another might register 120 mg/dL. This is still considered accurate by glucose meter manufacturers. One woman, who requested anonymity, noted differences between her own meter and the one used at the hospital where she delivered her son, now 2 weeks old.

"During delivery, I completely turned off my insulin pump and kept my sugars at 60 to 110 mg/dL throughout," she said. "The hospital insisted on using their meter, which was 20 percent lower than mine. So their meter said 60 and mine, with the same blood at the same time, would say 72. I just adjusted to their readings because they had to go by them."

Blood sugars can also affect when things get started. If your sugars are too high, a doctor may hold off on giving you Pitocin for an induction until you're back in range, Dr. Levy said.

Can I Eat Now? Do I Even Want To?

Once labor or your c-section begins, a dextrose drip can help treat a low blood sugar right away. If you're not on a drip, it's usually okay to drink some clear juice to treat a low blood sugar while you're in labor. Some hospital policies state that you cannot eat anything once you are in active labor, or the night before a scheduled c-section, or once an epidural or other anesthetic has been started. This is to reduce the chance that you will throw up food once the sedation has kicked in, which could cause you to choke to death or get an infection if tiny bits of food make their way into your lungs. Some hospitals allow you to drink fruit juice or have Popsicles to help bring your blood sugar up. "My perinatologist quietly told me it would probably be okay for me to treat a low the night before the surgery with 'something clear' to drink," said Katie, whose daughter arrived by planned c-section. "Thank goodness, because I was worried about how I would deal with a low when I wasn't supposed to eat after midnight. I ended up not being low, but it still was pretty awful not even being able to drink water." Check to see what the policy is about eating before delivering before you arrive to have your baby.

If your doctor gives you the okay to chow down, it's a good idea to eat something at home (or elsewhere, if you're out) if you have time before things gets started. "I made sure I ate a good, filling meal the night before my c-section," said Anna Tang Norton. "That held me until almost 24 hours later, when I was allowed to eat a liquid diet of broth, Jell-O, juice, milk, and water." Joy McCarren experienced something similar before being induced: "I was allowed to eat breakfast the day of my induction, and that helped to keep me stable throughout the day, since I wasn't allowed food after that." She delivered via cesarean two days after the induction was unsuccessful. "The morning of my c-section, I wasn't allowed to eat, but because of the dawn phenomenon, I didn't have trouble with low blood sugar." (The "dawn phenomenon" is when your body secretes hormones in the morning in response to waking up; it can cause blood sugars to increase in the mornings before you eat breakfast. Usually a pump basal adjustment or food choices before bed can help wrangle these early morning blood sugars.)[1]

If your labor goes on for a particularly long time, food intake can become an issue, as it did for Sara Bancroft. She was induced and was in labor for many hours before having a c-section. "I had some low blood sugars in the three days during my induction, mostly because [medical staff] would not let me eat anything," she said. "It was not easy managing diabetes on a liquid diet, and next time, I will insist on having food."

If your sugars are fine, noshing may be the last thing on your mind. "I wasn't told not to eat anything," said Amy Eddy, who was induced early in the morning and didn't start going into hard labor until well into the evening. "I remember having dinner, but that's when the pains really started, so dinner was no longer appetizing."

Then again, you may find you want food but your body has other ideas. Soon after my c-section, while in recovery, my stomach growled. Loudly. With a scheduled procedure, you're typically supposed to stop eating or drinking anything by midnight the night before, or six to eight hours beforehand. By the time I'd delivered my son, it had been more than half a day since I'd consumed anything. Whenever a nurse or doctor came toward my bed, I'd ask when I could eat. At one point, someone brought me a cup of ice chips, and I plowed through them. Sure enough, within an hour of my ice chip banquet, as I was chatting with my husband, the chips suddenly all came back up again— right onto the front of my hospital gown. Hello! What was that about? Clearly, my digestive system had different plans for me, though I was able to eat lightly several hours later and was back to a normal diet the next day.

Here We Go

So this is it—you're about to have your baby!

For my scheduled c-section, at week 37, day 6, I walked into the operating room and asked whether anyone had ever walked out. "It'd be a miracle, after having a spinal or epidural, if anyone could walk out," I was told. The anesthesia takes longer to wear off than a typical nonemergency cesarean lasts.

I got a spinal. To prepare for it, I was told to sit on the operating table, facing the side of the room, with my legs hanging down off the side of the bed, and to lean forward into the arms of a nurse standing in front of me. Getting an injection in the back would have freaked me out if I had thought about it too much, so I concentrated intently on the nurse I was leaning into ("You have very soft arms," I told her) and barely felt the needle at all. My legs and lower body felt really numb, really fast, and I wondered whether my blood sugar was dropping really quickly. It wasn't: I tested, and my blood sugar was pretty stable and had been in range all morning. Dave, attired in attractive scrubs and a really hip shower cap–like head covering, held my glucose meter and a camera throughout the process and stood by my side after I was already numbed and placed back on the operating table to lie down.

A ton of different medical people were in the room with Dave and me: the obstetrician, the anesthesiologist, a few nurses and residents, and a medical student (we were at a teaching hospital)—probably six or seven altogether. They introduced themselves before the procedure began. Then my obstetrician, who had cheerfully told me she loved delivering babies when I first walked into the room, got started. Someone draped a sheet up at my waist like a curtain so I couldn't see exactly what was happening, but I could feel pushing and pressing, and I soon smelled something burning. Normally, I ask plenty of questions, and when I asked whether I smelled something being cauterized, I was told yes. Did I want to know what was happening? I declined, in part because my husband doesn't want to know the gory details the way I like to (and he was right there), and in part because I didn't want to get scared or grossed out by anything *as it was happening*. I started to feel nauseous, and someone waved an alcohol swab under my nose, which immediately made me feel better. Suddenly my obstetrician yelled out, "I can see the head!" I asked why we couldn't hear anything, but within seconds we heard our baby crying loudly. "It's a boy!" our obstetrician announced, and she held him up over the sheet for us to see.

After our son, Ethan, had been cleaned up, weighed, and measured, the obstetrician handed him to Dave, while I was stitched up and the procedure was completed. (I wasn't allowed to hold the baby while I was still being worked on.) I felt nauseous again and asked, "Can I get more alcohol over here?" My obstetrician laughed and remarked, "No one's ever requested that during a c-section before." She then told me that I had beautiful fallopian tubes. Who knew?

Ethan's blood sugars were tested at birth and one hour, two hours, and five hours after he was born. Each test gave results in a normal range. For a baby, these numbers are typically lower than normal adult blood sugar ranges: newborn blood sugars of 40 to 70 mg/dL are considered normal, while a low at birth comes in around 20 to 30 mg/dL and is usually treated by breast-feeding or a bottle of formula, said nurse Mary Beth Bahren. "Low for the NICU means a blood sugar of zero to 20 mg/dL, or a newborn who doesn't respond to initial treatment for the first blood sugar reading at birth." Ask your doctor what the cutoff is for a low infant blood sugar at the place where you give birth.

Between my son's birth weight of 7 pounds, 9 ounces, and his blood sugars in the sixties, I was thrilled that he seemed to show none of the signs of macrosomia or hypoglycemia, and his Apgar scores were 8 and 9. He stayed with Dave or me for the rest of the day and never went to the NICU for anything. He looked great for a newborn, cried lustily, and slept nicely after being swaddled in a blanket and hat. Who could ask for more?

Apgar Explained

All infants are evaluated at one minute and five minutes of life for their Apgar scores.[2] These two scores measure five categories, each on a scale of 0 to 2: muscle tone, heart rate, breathing, reflexes, and color/appearance. Low numbers can indicate the need for immediate medical care at birth or shortly thereafter. Babies who score between 7 and 10 are typically considered healthy; numbers under 6 at one minute may mean the baby needs help breathing. Scores under 3 can necessitate lifesaving measures. At five minutes, a score of 7 to 10 is considered normal. Your doctor will tell you how to proceed next if your child scores under 6 at this point.

Experience and education can definitely help when it comes to handling subsequent pregnancies and deliveries. Michelle Kowalski was 39 weeks and 4 days along when she was induced with her third child (though it was only her first pregnancy with type 2 diabetes) and delivered vaginally. "I was induced mainly because I was taking blood thinners [not related to diabetes] and my doctor wanted to be in control of that," she said. "Of all my kids, this was the best experience—if only I could have had the third kid first! I knew what to expect, I knew how to push, and I felt more in control."

Kowalski had discussed with her CDE how to handle her insulin and food intake before her induction, and she was given Pitocin at 5:30 a.m. the day she delivered. She ate a light breakfast of natural peanut butter on high-fiber bread with water. She had been splitting her long-acting doses of insulin by this point in her pregnancy, and injected half the amount of her long-acting insulin the night before and did not take a shot of rapid-acting insulin for the meal. "I hoped the protein and carbs would sustain my blood sugar throughout the birth," she said. "My plan was a little thrown off because I had taken my evening dose of long-acting insulin too late the night before and decided to wait until I got to the hospital to take the morning dose. When I got to the hospital, the nurses advised me not to take the [other half of the long-acting insulin that morning], so I listened. It turned out to be a good idea as my sugar stayed under 110 for the whole process, including laboring for five hours."

Kowalski's daughter had a blood sugar of 28 mg/dL at birth, which "freaked me out, but the nurse reminded me that a baby's blood sugar typically runs much lower than an adult's, and that while 28 was low, it wasn't the same as if I was 28." The baby breast-fed and drank some formula, which brought her blood sugar up to 50 mg/dL, which is considered normal. The baby did not need to go to the NICU and was otherwise born healthy.

Other mothers mentioned problems with medications administered during labor or a c-section. "I was induced at 38 or 39 weeks, per my doctor's standard protocol, and everything seemed okay to me," said Amy Eddy. "The only thing was that the drugs made me very sleepy well into the next day. I was even too sleepy to want to hold my son right after he was born—I told them to give him to my husband first." Sharon was induced at 38 weeks and 5 days, but some things never came together. "I was supposed to have Cervidil [a vaginal suppository that softens the cervix and prepares the body for labor and delivery] the night before, but they had no room [at the hospital] until 3 a.m.," she said. "I opted to go then, but I didn't get an IV inserted until 5 a.m. By then, the doctor decided to skip the Cervidil and go straight to Pitocin. I never progressed. By noon we decided, as we'd discussed ahead of time, to not make this a long labor that ended in a c-section anyway and to just do it while all the docs we wanted were around." Her daughter arrived via cesarean that day.

"Obviously, the outcome was amazing, but the only thing I wished had gone differently was that I was so doped up that I couldn't really appreciate it," she said. "I am apparently very sensitive to medications and was rather out of it during the delivery and for about an hour afterward. I plan to try harder for less medication or none for the epidural next time." Her daughter was taken to the hospital's nursery for three hours without Sharon or her husband and was fed an ounce of formula to treat a borderline low blood sugar. "We were not told or asked about this," she said. "We plan on being more forceful with future children—only letting the doctors do things we aren't comfortable with if the child's health is clearly in jeopardy."

Traicy Lewis had a different issue: her drugs weren't administered early enough. "My son's arrival was unexpected because he came at 35 weeks," she said. "My labor was somewhat fast—four hours total. I think it was faster than they anticipated, and it caught them off guard. They had problems getting IVs in, because my veins are deep, and they couldn't get the epidural in. I was eight centimeters dilated after the third try with the epidural, and my doctor came in and said, 'Why wasn't this already done?'" Lewis's son was breech, something she knew already, but she had hoped the baby would turn on his own. Because of his early arrival, which was not attributed to Lewis's diabetes, the baby didn't turn in time. She ultimately delivered a healthy baby boy by emergency c-section.

Some women said that parts of the experience were frightening. Heidi Wickstrom and her doctor wanted her to deliver vaginally because of the doctor's concerns about healing poorly after a c-section. When she developed high blood pressure, she took Pitocin to induce at 39 weeks but had a tough labor. She began pushing at 6 p.m., 11 hours after taking the Pitocin. "My daughter was getting stuck due to her size: 8 pounds, 9 ounces," she said. "After one hour of pushing, my doctor tried the vacuum with no luck, and then forceps. I had pushed for an hour and a half when my doctor told me, 'One more push with forceps, or it's a c-section,' and she came out. I had horrible tears, but everyone was okay. It was scary and difficult. If and when I get pregnant again, I am pretty sure I will just go for a c-section."

Others said they were lucky to have a terrific experience and wouldn't change a thing. "It was absolutely amazing," said Yehudit W., who delivered vaginally at close to 40 weeks. She worked with a doula, midwife, and perinatologist and wanted to deliver as naturally as possible, with minimal intervention. "I wanted to be there and be able to take part in the birth process. Working together with my body was crucial: mobility at all stages of labor was extremely important, and I was aiming to avoid having an epidural as well as any other unnecessary medical interventions." Because she hadn't started active labor on her own after several hours, Yehudit took small amounts of Pitocin under her midwife's guidance. Things moved forward, and six hours later her daughter was born. "I was thrilled that I was able to physically, emotionally, and spiritually be there during the birth and afterwards," she said. "I took care of my insulin needs, but had my husband and doula around if it became difficult for me. I wear a pump. My sugars were normal with occasional lows during my labor, and I was able to drink apple juice to counter the lows. I checked my own sugars with the help of my husband and doula."

Elizabeth Edelman also spoke highly of having her baby. "I had a natural birth and things went 100 percent according to plan," she said. "I was surprised that it happened that easily, and I know I'm very lucky to be able to say this. My labor was fast, four hours, and relatively easy." She was attached to a fetal monitor when she arrived at the hospital, at 4 centimeters dilated and at 39 weeks and a few days, but when the monitor didn't show any fetal problems, she was allowed to take it off and go into a shower to help speed things up.

"I just breathed through it," she said. "The deep breathing is paramount if you're planning a natural birth. I loved being in the shower while in labor and sat on one of those exercise balls in the shower and rocked back and forth with the water on my belly. I was able to turn inward and I didn't want anyone around. My husband and our doula were in the bathroom with me, but left me alone. I went from 4 centimeters, which is where I was at when we arrived at the hospital, to 10 centimeters in an hour. If you're planning a natural birth, I highly recommend the shower. It's heavenly! And if that's the route you want to take, just know that it can be done with diabetes!"

Edelman wore her insulin pump most of the time and was able to check her blood sugars herself. "My water broke at 3 a.m., when I was asleep, and when I checked my sugar, it was normal," she said. "It was around 200 at the end of labor, only because I disconnected for an hour and sat in the shower at the hospital. Once I delivered, I took a correction for the high and was right back to normal. My husband was also aware of what to do, and my endo had a set of instructions if the nurses needed to intervene."

Edelman's daughter was born healthy and had no low blood sugars anytime after the birth. Edelman herself was delighted with how things turned out. "I wouldn't have changed one thing about my birth experience," she said. "It was amazing."

What Happens Next?

Enjoy your new arrival. The day you give birth will hopefully be filled with terrific memories and experiences. You've done a boatload of work to get to this point—sit back and relax. As soon as your baby is born, he or she will typically be evaluated using the Apgar test, cleaned up, given an identification bracelet and anklet, treated with an eye ointment to avoid infection, diapered, and swaddled to keep warm. This is also when the baby's blood sugar is first checked, typically by taking blood from the heel. If your baby is going to need to go to the NICU, it will likely happen now, but definitely find out what circumstances might require a NICU visit. For many healthy babies born to moms with diabetes, there will likely be no medical reason for a NICU stay. Other babies show signs of needing extra help at birth, and sometimes a NICU visit is needed. Delivery before term can mean your baby's lungs or other organs are not fully developed. Sometimes low blood sugars don't respond to immediate treatment.

"I was not happy with the after-the-birth experience because I did not get correct or accurate information, and that stressed me out," said Alycia Green. Her son was breech, and Green delivered by a scheduled c-section at 39 weeks. His blood sugars were too low at birth—around 30 mg/dL—and Green was not able to see her son right away. He was taken to the NICU for immediate treatment with a pacifier dipped into a glucose solution, and he was fed formula, which Green said she had not wanted. While she was recovering from her c-section, Green's nurse called the NICU and Green expected that her son would be brought back to her. Instead, the nurse returned to her room empty-handed and said the formula and pacifier treatments had been insufficient; the baby had had to be given an IV to raise his blood sugar levels.

"I felt so horrible," said Green. "I had excellent control throughout the pregnancy and did not anticipate any big problems. I don't feel that I was properly prepared or informed by my OB about what would probably happen, so I was very upset. They wheeled me into the NICU to see my son for a mere five minutes, then I went to my room. He couldn't be with me the entire first night because of the IV and sugar issue."

Green said the doctors and nurses on staff never gave her a solid explanation why her son's sugars went so low or why they didn't rise after the initial treatment. "My numbers were in the normal range prior to delivery," she said. "[My doctors] had me on both an insulin and a glucose drip, and I wasn't paying much attention to what my numbers were during delivery. While in recovery, my sugars were in the 200s, which led me to believe, and I still believe to this day, that

I might not have been getting the proper ratio of insulin to glucose. [My husband and I also] realized that I was being given IV antibiotics that were in a glucose solution. My husband actually caught that—the pharmacy, the nurses, and the doctors did not. Once that issue was resolved, the numbers started coming under control again."

In addition, Green's son initially tested positive for a mandatory MRSA check given to all babies in the NICU, although his reading was eventually determined to have been a false positive. (MRSA, short for methicillin-resistant *Staphylococcus aureus*, is a potentially fatal strain of a staph bacterial infection that is resistant to common antibiotic treatment.)[3] However, her son was kept in isolation because of the original false positive. Green herself later spiked a fever, which kept her out of the NICU and prolonged the separation between her and her son. "Basically, I gave birth to my son at 12:36 p.m. on Tuesday and did not get him in my hospital room until Friday evening," she said. "Due to all the circumstances, I only saw him for about 40 minutes during that time. I know the MRSA and the fever issue weren't diabetes related, but I still feel extreme guilt that I was the cause of him having to be placed in the NICU in the first place. I feel if he hadn't been taken there, then I would have had him sooner. The entire experience was so gut wrenching that I am still disturbed about the entire hospital stay to this day."

The experience taught her to be more assertive in the future. "Next time, I plan on being a bigger pain in the butt," she said, "asking tons of questions and not taking 'I don't know' as an answer."

Tips for a NICU Stay

If a newborn needs to go to an intensive care unit for close observation or medical care, the situation can be stressful for any parent. Here's some insight from women who have been there:

- Speak up. "Don't be afraid to ask questions," said Katrina Holm. "If you don't understand what the doctor is telling you, ask again. Carry a notebook around and write down questions as you think about them. When the doctor answers you, write down their answer so you can go back and look at it later. You will not remember everything they tell you." It's not a bad idea to turn up the friendliness factor for the NICU staff, even if you are stressed or scared and the last thing you feel like doing is being nice to anyone. "Befriend the NICU nurses as much as possible, and try to know the nurses by name," said Alycia Green. "I found that I was able to get more information from the nurses, and in a more timely manner, than from the doctors." Be organized about taking notes. "Keep track of the date, time, names, and responses you receive when inquiring about the care of your baby," Green said.

- Capture the moments. These are your baby's first days, weeks, or months, and there's no reason not to memorialize them just because he or she is in the NICU. "Ask if you can bring a camera to take pictures of your baby," said Holm. "Also ask the nurse if you can leave a disposable camera, and when they give the baby a bath or other tasks, if they would mind taking a quick picture of your baby. These will be cherished memories, even though it seems silly at the time."

- Trust yourself. You are your baby's mother, and if you are spending a lot of time in the NICU with your child, you will know his or her habits and patterns better than anyone else. "If you see something that you think isn't working, or that you think would work better, don't be afraid to bring ideas forward and to be fairly firm on them," said Bethany Rose, whose daughter spent time in the immediate care nursery, which was one step down from her hospital's NICU. Her daughter initially had feeding problems, but Rose noticed that some solutions (such as swaddling) worked better than others (such as letting the baby pace herself while eating). She and her husband talked to the nursing staff about how the baby ate, and they developed a list of feeding instructions that the nurses followed when Rose and her husband were not in the immediate care nursery with their daughter. "Our input was valuable in getting [our daughter] to overcome some of her difficulties and come home to us," she said.

- Practice self-care. You're likely exhausted, and you just gave birth. Give yourself time to heal and rest, particularly if you delivered by cesarean. This applies to your time in the hospital and when you go home if you need to leave your child in the NICU for care. "Some people will make you feel like you need to spend every waking hour at the hospital with your baby, but you don't," said Rose. "You need to do what's best for you. It is important to make sure you get enough rest to make sure that you are in good shape when you baby comes home." Adequate rest also helps with milk production if you're planning to breast-feed. "Do what you have to do—you'll have plenty of time to bond when [your baby] comes home," she said.

- You're bound to bond. There's a notion that you need to bond with your child immediately after giving birth by spending a lot of time breast-feeding and laying the baby on your chest for skin-to-skin contact, among other things. These are all great if you can do them, but if you can't because your baby had to go immediately to the NICU, it does not mean you'll never be close to your child. You have a lifetime, and certainly enough time while your baby is in fact still a baby, to deepen your connection to one another. "I was very nervous that I wouldn't bond with my son because he was in the NICU and I was pumping breast milk to take to him all the time, and he wasn't getting a lot of contact time with me," said Anna Tang Norton. "But I figured out how to hold him, coddle him, and talk to him, and we bonded immediately. My husband did the same. He would visit during bath times, changed diapers, held him, and so on. We made the most out of a difficult situation." She also invited other family members to see her son, as the NICU rules allowed. "Initially, we didn't want our family to visit him, but on the second day, we realized that the comfort of family and friends was as important as the medical attention he received," she said. "Naturally we were careful and followed NICU protocol, but we saw him often and we spoke to him and coddled him."

- Enjoy the time. "Try to include some fun activities in your day, either when you're away from the hospital, or even at the hospital when your baby is sleeping," said Rose. "Remember: He or she has the best babysitters money can buy right now, so take advantage. Go for picnic lunches, see a movie, visit a friend, indulge in a good book—anything to break up the day and provide a pleasant distraction." The NICU stay is usually only a short visit and ultimately a very small part of your family's life. "I would tell parents not to stress about the NICU," said Norton. "In many ways, it's more attentive than the well-baby nursery. My son had two nurses at all times and was constantly tended to. I had no problems knowing he was in their care."

What Changes for You: Medications

Immediately after you give birth, your insulin needs will change, usually plummeting to what they were before you got pregnant, or even less. Work with your endo to figure out how much insulin you will need and how your insulin-to-carb ratios will change, rather than figuring it out on your own. "There's no guarantee that what amount of insulin you needed to take before is what you'll need now," Dr. Carol Levy said. "There's a weight shift and usually breast-feeding going on. Typically, I will tell patients to take 50 percent of what they were taking during pregnancy, and then follow them depending on what happens. I give them their postdelivery insulin rates—what I predict they will be—ahead of time, so while they're in labor, they can set another profile on their pumps so they don't have to worry about it when they're exhausted after labor." Other endocrinologists do things differently and might recommend halving your pre-pregnancy insulin rates once you give birth. Physicians have their own methods of determining what your post-pregnancy insulin doses should be; ask your doctor the reasoning behind the doses chosen for your immediate postpartum care.

As mentioned earlier, you won't shed all your pregnancy weight immediately, and the extra pounds can affect how much insulin you need right away. And breast-feeding, which is discussed in further detail in Chapter 8, burns a lot of calories and glucose. If you're nursing, you'll notice right away that you need far less insulin (and more snacks or glucose sources within reach while feeding your baby) than you did before.

Other medications that you stopped or changed when you found out you were pregnant may be re-prescribed after you give birth. Your doctor may recommend that you stay off some meds if you are breast-feeding. If you take a pill for a thyroid disorder, such as levothyroxine, Synthroid, or Levoxyl, the dose will likely change throughout pregnancy, and you will probably return to your preconception dose right after you have your baby. Statins, on the other hand, which help treat high cholesterol, are not recommended for breast-feeding mothers because they can cross into breast milk and affect your baby's system. If you are type 2 and treated your diabetes with pills before becoming pregnant, talk to your doctor about whether you will return to oral meds or stay on insulin, particularly if you are nursing.

"It's critical to follow up with your regular endocrinologist, ophthalmologist, and/or nephrologist as soon as you can after giving birth and resume taking any meds you may have been taken off during pregnancy and lactation," said Suzie Won, who had kidney issues going into pregnancy and was especially concerned about resuming medications that preserved her kidney function while she nursed her daughter for 15 months.

Handling your own health needs while managing the day-to-day details of raising a new baby becomes a whole new balancing act. With a lot of planning, support, and, in some cases, relaxed standards, you can totally do it. Rock on, Mom!

8

The New Mom, With Diabetes

Congratulations! Now the juggling really begins, because suddenly you're responsible not just for yourself but also for your newborn son or daughter. Balancing your own health needs with those of your child is the hallmark of parenting with diabetes. For now, consider how you'll handle your diabetes care, along with new parenthood issues, for the first crazy few weeks. If you're breast-feeding, you might experience low blood sugars. If you're formula feeding, will your history with diabetes influence which type of formula you'll use? It's also important to recognize the signs of postpartum depression, particularly as people with diabetes are more likely to deal with depression anyway. Then come the issues that any new mom deals with: sleeping (or not), exercising (or not), going back to work (or not), and more. Finally, think about options for birth control; someday you'll be ready to get down with your partner again (even if most of the time you're just trying to get down for a solid nap when you can).

Mothering With Diabetes: The Early Days

The hospital gave you the go-ahead to leave with your baby, and now you and your partner are on your own. In the midst of installing the car seat properly, dressing the baby, and hauling home all the swag (newborn gifts, free parenting magazines, coupons for diaper cream, whatever else you scored, the car seat bucket, and, oh yeah, the baby), you may forget to test your blood sugar or think about the numbers. And for the first time in more than nine months, you may not stress out right away if your sugars stray above 140 mg/dL.

This can be both freeing and disconcerting. On one hand, your blood sugars probably weren't as tight before pregnancy as they were while you were pregnant. A high reading isn't great in the long run for any of us, but the reality is that out-of-range numbers on the higher side don't typically make you feel so terrible that you must treat them immediately. Sometimes they just happen. If my baby is wailing from exhaustion and my sugar is, say, 160 mg/dL, I know I'm going to soothe my baby first and bolus later. Sometimes, in the crush of these early days and nights, it can be hard to remember whether your sugar is where it is because you just ate and your sugars should be coming down after the food and insulin get through you or because you forgot to take insulin for breakfast three hours ago—particularly if you're facing a diaper blowout that requires a lot of cleanup. (And where's that extra package of wipes when you need it?) As tough as it is, try not to let the average of your blood sugars soar once you get home and are settling in. Keep an eye on things when you can.

"It's hard," said Nicole Ishikawa, 31, type 1, of Lawrence, Kansas. Her son is 5 months old. "Managing my blood sugars is no longer on my top five priority list. I no longer have the time to test every two hours, cook healthy meals, come up with a creative meal plan, and so on."

Focusing on diabetes care can be tough even when your kid grows out of the newborn stage. "Once I had my baby, I stopped taking such meticulous care of myself," said Amy Eddy. "Three years later, I'm still in the same patterns and bad habits, though I'm trying to change. Try to continue the same healthy patterns and habits you were on while you were pregnant, even though it's easy to say 'Yay, I don't have to worry about it anymore!' because really, you do. You want to make sure you are at your best physically and mentally so you can take good care of that baby. If you aren't taking care of you, you won't be at your best."

Use whatever technology is available. "I highly recommend a CGM system for new mothers on the pump," said Bethany Rose. "In the first few weeks after my daughter was born, I had a couple of very low blood sugars while I was getting used to my new insulin needs. When I'm sleep deprived and distracted, I often don't notice my blood sugar dropping as fast as when I'm more 'with it.' When my husband's at work, I really don't want to risk any scary lows. The CGM is great for providing me with that security."

If a CGM is out of your budget and your insurance company won't budge on coverage, going low-tech can still help you remember to test frequently. "When you are busy taking care of kids, it's easy to forget to test your sugar," said Clemma Muller. "Set alarms during the day, if necessary, to help you remember to test regularly." If you have an insulin pump, it may have alarms, but setting a clock can work just as well.

Your body is handling things differently than it was when you were pregnant, and even before you were pregnant, so frequent testing can help you figure out what is going on and why. "Check your blood sugars often," said Dr. Tamara Takoudes. "Check during breast-feeding, check when you eat, check when you can. Keep a snack available when you are breast-feeding, as this is when you may go low. It is most important to check, even though the control does not need to be as tight as it was now that the baby is out. But if you are not checking, you cannot make adjustments to know how to improve or what is happening or changing with your new self."

In addition to testing, make sure you can treat your lows quickly. It can be tough to take the time to test and treat a low if your baby is screaming from HUNGER!NOW!, but you've gotta take care of you. Let your kid get a lung workout while you chug some juice. "You must treat yourself first if you have a low," said Abby Nagel, who said she felt guilty and wanted to ignore her own needs when her daughter cried or needed something. "I have learned to tell her that 'Mommy is low and needs to drink some juice, and then I will be right there to help her.' Now, six years later, she and her 3-year-old sister are very aware when Mommy is low and are pretty good natured about waiting a few minutes before I get to either of them."

It's a great idea to build up your glucose supplies before you give birth so you can easily treat low blood sugars once you're home with your infant. Buy a case or two of juice boxes from a wholesale store or have someone bring you a load of glucose tabs or LifeSavers or your treatment of choice to ensure that you won't be stuck without a sugar stash. (Stock up when sales are on. For years, my mom bought me holiday packages of LifeSavers immediately after Christmas or Valentine's Day, typically for a tiny fraction of the usual price. Months later, I'd tear off candy wrappers with snow or hearts so that I could inhale six candies to treat a low.)

"Don't be afraid to ask for help," said Anna Tang Norton. "Transitioning into motherhood is tough, let alone adding diabetes into the equation." You may be used to handling your diabetes on your own—really, how long did you do this before you got pregnant?—but having to deal with a newborn might throw a wrench into your system. It's definitely not embarrassing or a failure for you to reach out for assistance. Ask someone to bring over a freezer-friendly meal so that you don't have to cook on top of everything else, or have a friend stock up your shelves by doing a grocery run while you're at home.

"It can be daunting juggling a new baby and diabetes, but it certainly can be done," said Joy McCarren. "Once you establish a routine, it becomes second nature. Others may not understand the extra load you are carrying, being a diabetic parent, but if they are willing to help out in any way, accept the help. Don't become discouraged, and do not compare yourself to other moms who are not diabetic. We deal with a whole different set of responsibilities and issues that most people cannot understand. It will not always be easy, but it is manageable. Just take it one day, or one hour, or one minute at a time."

Healing After a Vaginal or Cesarean Delivery

No matter how you gave birth, there's likely some recovering to do. If you had tears during a vaginal delivery, an episiotomy, or a cesarean delivery, part of you was stitched up or stapled closed and the wound needs to heal. If your blood sugars are high, the process can be slower and you can be more prone to infection (as is typical with any cut or blemish with diabetes, anyway).

"Incision healing is affected adversely with a long labor prior to a cesarean delivery, a repeat cesarean, and/or poor glucose control—say, over 200 mg/dL, often—in the postpartum period," said Dr. Tamara Takoudes.[1] Her research found that women with pre-existing diabetes are two and a half times more likely to have problems with wound healing after a cesarean delivery, including such complications as wound infection, wound separation wider than 1 centimeter, or wounds bursting open after being surgically closed. Trying to maintain normal blood sugars while handling a newborn's needs is tough, but returning to the doctor's office regularly because your wound is infected or leaking who knows what all over your underwear is not something you want to deal with if you don't have to. Keep an eye on your sugars so that your incisions can close up properly.

If you're in any pain, there's no reason to suffer. Some medications are safe to use if you are breast-feeding, and they shouldn't have any effect on your blood sugar control. "Pain itself can cause disruption in blood glucose, so controlling it is most important," said nurse Mary Beth Bahren. Taking meds for pain won't necessarily make you loopy, either; the drugs are to help you feel normal, not euphoric or out of it. Talk to your doc about pharmaceutical side effects to see whether one prescription or over-the-counter medication is better for you than another.

For other medical issues during pregnancy or postpartum, check with your doctor about which meds are okay for you to take. "I had two c-sections and two easy recoveries," said Katrine Whiteson, 31, type 1, of Geneva, Switzerland. Her kids are 2 years and 4 months old. Her first c-section was done after 36 hours of labor, pushing, and an infection, and the second happened after she was diagnosed with a severe form of pre-eclampsia that caused liver bruising. "I wasn't able to use ibuprofen after having pre-eclampsia, and I still did not have much discomfort with only Tylenol after the anesthetic wore off," she said. Walking helped her heal. "Both times, I did not have serious discomfort after just a day or two. I was walking around the next day, and I felt pretty much completely myself after a week or two. I often went for long walks after the first week or so, which helped me recover and surprised some of my friends who weren't able to do that after more straightforward birth experiences."

All About Breast-Feeding

Newborns eat often. Frequent feedings define babyhood, and even though I'd heard this before giving birth, the reality of it was something else. Feeding my newborn son was for me hands down the toughest thing about becoming a new parent. The lack of sleep, the diaper changing, the crying, the spitting up, the fussiness, the need to change all the soiled clothes (both mine and my kid's)—it all pales in comparison when I think about the efforts I made to feed my kid directly from the boob. Frustrating doesn't even begin to cover it.

No matter how you decide to feed your baby, you will hear, again and again, that breast milk is the best food you can give your child. According to the National Women's Health Information Center, a division of the U.S. Department of Health and Human Services, "breast milk has antibodies that help protect babies from germs, illness, and even SIDS [sudden infant death syndrome].[2] Breast-feeding is linked to a lower risk in infants for developing type 1 and type 2 diabetes, ear infections, stomach viruses, diarrhea, respiratory infections, asthma, obesity, childhood leukemia, and other health problems. Mothers who breast-feed have a lower risk of developing breast cancer, ovarian cancer, and postpartum depression."

Because breast-fed infants have a lower risk of developing diabetes, I really wanted to nurse and feed my son breast milk. People also mentioned how easy it was, how you didn't need to wash bottles and nipples, how you could instantly soothe a crying baby without having to prepare a bottle of formula, and how cheap breast-feeding was compared with formula feeding. Plus, the stuff comes directly from you—how much more natural can you get?

Nursing was none of those things for me. After I had spent a small fortune on nursing tank tops and bras, two lactation consultants, a breast pump and accessories, two hands-free pumping bras, and lactation-boosting herbs and medications, my otherwise happy son would let me know he was hungry by crying or stuffing his whole hand into his mouth. He would latch on to me, look like he was feeding, and sound like he was swallowing; after it seemed like he'd been eating for an eternity—far longer than I was told a nursing session should take—I'd take him off the breast... and he'd scream.

It turns out my kid was hungry. On day three of his life, a nurse at the hospital told me he had lost more than 10 percent of his body weight. This is a sign that a baby isn't getting enough to eat and something needs to change.

The nurse told me I'd have to start giving my son formula in addition to my breast-feeding efforts. I was not happy about this at all—wasn't breast milk the best thing for my kid, the Whole Foods of nutrition? And wasn't there some link between formula feeding and developing type 1 diabetes? The idea of giving my son something that might trigger type 1 diabetes for him made me panic and kept me committed to trying to nurse or pump breast milk for as long as I could.

Reluctantly, I added formula feeding to the mix, choosing a formula where the milk proteins were hydrolyzed (broken down into the smallest pieces possible). These brands are typically used for colicky babies, but I figured it might be a way to ward off potential problems that drinking cow's milk protein could cause for a baby with a possible genetic link to diabetes. Notice all the potentials here: my husband and I spent a lot of extra money to buy this stuff for something I worried about but couldn't prove because of ongoing studies. For me, the peace of mind was worth it. You, like many other women with diabetes who did not freak out about formula choice the way I did, may think differently.

Now that I had a formula chosen, it was time to feed my son. Because I was still trying to nurse, I worried that feeding my kid with a bottle might make him refuse the breast, as a bottle nipple works a lot faster. Dave and I began finger feeding, a technique that uses a syringe and tubing taped to one's finger. This process added more steps to what was already a long and complex system. I was now trying to nurse for a long while, finger feeding formula, pumping to get any extra milk out of me to stimulate my body to *Make more milk!*, and then washing out everything and looking at the clock to see when my kid might need to eat again.

Needless to say, nursing stressed me out. For all the effort I put into it, with the pre-nurse breast massaging, the nipple shield, the prescription nipple ointment to prevent pain and infection, the increased water intake, and the positioning, my son never seemed satisfied. A week later, an expensive lactation consultant confirmed the problem. She watched me pump, told me I had a low milk supply, and said I should consider breast milk to be the dessert, not the main meal, for my son. She also said I could quit with the finger feeding and move on to bottles, already. Doing so, thankfully, didn't make a bit of difference with my son's latching, but it did make the overall process easier.

I'd already started taking fenugreek, an herbal supplement sold over the counter that is supposed to boost milk supply for lactating women. I later upped the dose, and when that didn't help, I tried Reglan and Domperidone, two prescription medications that can help increase milk supply. They have worked for many women; sadly, for me they never did enough.

Because nursing wasn't enjoyable, it was much easier for me to pump (and see exactly how much I could produce) than to sit for hours trying to nurse and wonder whether my son would ever be satiated or whether I would ever feel like I knew what I was doing. I gave up breast-feeding after about five weeks but pumped breast milk for eight and a half months, until my already diminished supply just gave out. Ethan drank hydrolyzed formula until his first birthday.

I never got a solid explanation for why my supply was low and why nursing was such a bust for me. There are theories about diabetes and low supply, cesarean deliveries, and advanced maternal age, but I couldn't find anything definitive. Was it genetic? Related to diabetes? The result of having a scheduled c-section? Something else? Who knows. Hopefully, you will have a much easier time if you want to nurse. I am clearly not representative of most women with diabetes who want to breast-feed. Many moms are able to do it and adore it.

"I am still breast-feeding my 9-month-old," said Elizabeth Edelman. "I love it. Just take a deep breath in, and enjoy the time with your new baby."

Breast-feeding helps you lose weight and lowers your blood sugars because it churns through so many calories and carbs. This is great if you're trying to shed excess pregnancy weight but requires some planning (in terms of having glucose handy and lowering your insulin doses) to make sure you're not dropping low while your starving child just got comfortable. Eating something before a nursing session or keeping snacks nearby can help prevent you from bottoming out while your babe is on the boob.

"Having low blood sugar while caring for an infant is *very* stressful," said Suzie Won, who breast-fed for 15 months. "Be sure to have plenty of juice boxes, candy, nutrition bars and other forms of sugar that you can reach, even while nursing or rocking baby to sleep. Capri Sun makes 100-percent fruit juice pouches, which are a life saver for me. When the baby is crying, and I'm flustered because my sugar is low, I try not to forget to treat my low blood sugar; it's easy to get distracted by a screaming baby. Put baby back in her crib and be sure to back up the simple sugar with protein and fat, especially when nursing, because it really does lower your blood sugars. Drink tons of water and fluids to replace what the body has taken to produce breast milk."

Others noted that the process can be affected as the child grows. "I had always planned on breast-feeding, mainly because I knew the health benefits for the baby, and also because I wanted that bonding time with my child," said Joy McCarren, who nursed for 14 months. "It was somewhat of a roller coaster ride. Just when I thought I had things figured out, my daughter would go through a growth spurt, and my milk production would change, causing my sugars to become unpredictable again. I found that it was often an hour or two after breast-feeding that I would notice a sudden drop in my blood sugars, not necessarily right while I was breast-feeding. I found that eating high-protein, high-fiber foods helped to keep me stabilized. Also, eating small snacks throughout the day worked well."

While breast-feeding has been shown to lower blood sugars, what happens if you start nursing when your sugars are high? The majority of endocrinologists, obstetricians, and pediatricians don't have a problem with this, and will tell you to go right ahead. However, there is a school of thought that nursing should be avoided while blood sugars are too high. Lois Jovanovič, MD, FACE, the chief executive officer and chief scientific officer of the Sansum Diabetes Research Institute in Santa Barbara, California, said that breast milk changes when a mother's blood sugar levels rise above 150 mg/dL. The extra glucose makes the milk taste sweeter. "Babies fed sugary milk are irritable, hungry, always crying between meals, and can't go more than 1½ hours between meals," she said. "They're having reactive hyperglycemia. If you're breast-feeding, the milk has to be normal."

If you test your blood sugar and find you're above a normal range, Dr. Jovanovič recommends pumping and discarding the milk and feeding your child with a bottle of previously pumped milk that was obtained when your sugars were in range. "Keep a fresh bottle of milk in the fridge, so you don't have to feed the baby milk that is too sweet," she said.

This may be a process of trial and error for you. With my low supply, the idea of pumping and dumping breast milk would have horrified me. And once my kid was actually fed, sometimes with enough breast milk for one meal, he was cheerful, so I didn't see the ill effects of sweet milk. But Suzie Won, who saw Dr. Jovanovič as part of a research study while Won was pregnant, followed the guidelines. "I also learned from Dr. Jovanovič that when mom's blood sugar is [high], the excess sugar spills into breast milk, causing baby to vomit," she said. "I did notice this happening, so we continued to supplement with formula when it was necessary, but primarily relied on nursing. My milk supply seemed to increase when my blood sugars ran high. I would 'pump and dump' when my blood sugars were too high, and even the act of pumping reliably helped bring my blood sugars down."

Breast-feeding and pumping breast milk are skills that require a lot of practice. There are techniques for latching, positioning, and so on that go beyond the scope of this book. Talk to the lactation consultants in the hospital where you deliver, consult any friends and family who have successfully breast-fed, and seek support from associations or nearby groups that are all about breast-feeding and pumping. "In order to help nursing, immerse yourself with other moms who were successful, and do not talk to people (mothers, sisters, or friends) who say, 'I tried it and it was too hard,' as this is very negative and not helpful for you," said Dr. Tamara Takoudes. "Low milk supply can sometimes be associated with type 2 diabetes, or polycystic ovarian disease, but this should never discourage anyone from trying as there are ways to try to maximize milk supply even if this does happen. You will never know unless you try."

While you may not have access to the extended families and villages of yesteryear filled with helpful female elders, consider this collection of advice if you're learning to breast-feed or pump breast milk. (See the Resources section for links to more hands-on help, too.)

- "You may be in some pain the first few days, and it may have nothing to do with a latching problem," said Yehudit W., who is still nursing her 9-month-old. "Sometimes, your body just needs to toughen up and get acclimated, and it may take a couple of days or so for this to take effect."

- "I wanted to nurse for various reasons, and tried it several times in the hospital," said Katie. She is still breast-feeding her 7-month-old daughter, who was born by c-section and went to the NICU for three days. "I pumped the colostrum [the liquid you produce at birth before your actual milk comes in; colostrum is full of antibodies and minerals] the day of delivery, instead of feeding it directly to my daughter, because she was in the NICU."

- "You just have to keep at it," said Michelle Kowalski, who breast-fed her youngest daughter for 17 months and her two older kids for 4 to 6 months. "With my third, I had incredibly sore nipples, and it was very, very painful when she latched on, but I was determined to get through it, so I kept at it. I think to be the most successful, you have to shun bottles, you have to be the one to get up with the baby in the middle of the night, and if you want to be successful long term, the baby has to nurse all the time. Let the baby get used to mom, and if you have to give a bottle, really limit it."

- "Educate yourself ahead of time and get good support—it is the most important thing," said Clemma Muller, who has concurrently nursed one son for 3½ years and another son for 14 months. "Moms and babies must learn how to breast-feed and it isn't always natural or easy. If you do not have any local relatives or friends with experience, contact La Leche League or Attachment Parenting International or find their online communities [see Resources]. Regardless of whether you agree or disagree with their philosophies, both organizations are strongly dedicated to supporting nursing families. Last tip: Lanolin cream will save your life in the first four weeks. Apply it to the nipples after *every* feeding to prevent chapping and cuts. You will still have some pain, but by four weeks or so it will get better."

- "When I was low, it was more difficult to let down [eject breast milk], I think," said Sharon, who breast-fed for 23 months. "I was nervous while nursing with high blood sugars, initially, but my pediatrician convinced me it was fine. Don't let potential problems go on, as they are easier to fix sooner. There are many free nursing support groups run through hospitals, La Leche League, and other breast-feeding support programs that are great for learning tips and staying connected with other new moms."

- "You will need help, and it's best to look for help in advance," said Nicole Ishikawa, who is nursing her 3-month-old. "Get to know lactation consultants, maybe a postpartum doula, a breast-feeding support group, or friends who have nursed successfully. It's good to have a few phone numbers you can call on the first day home (or after weeks!) when nothing works and you need someone to come over and help."

- "I started breast-feeding at about five weeks," said Bethany Rose, whose daughter was in an intermediate care nursery for three weeks, in part because of feeding difficulties. She has breast-fed for four and a half months. "[My daughter] started off being tube fed and then bottle fed. I pumped, though, and she was on solely breast milk within the second week of her life. The transition was tricky because she was so used to the bottle nipple. A lactation consultant suggested using a nipple shield to bridge the gap between bottle nipple and human nipple, and it's worked like a charm. I really recommend using one for moms who are having trouble switching from bottle to breast. Also, I spent a lot of time trying to increase my milk production after the c-section, to the point that my supply was much greater than my daughter's demand. When we switched to breast-feeding, I had to strategically pump a little bit less because if I just stopped pumping altogether, I would get very sore and end up with blocked milk ducts. Try to match the pumping to the baby's demand by pumping for less time at each pumping session, rather than trying to pump as much milk as possible. It's great to have a lot of milk, but it's not so great to have painful, full breasts!"

- "I think breast-feeding made me nervous, which made for erratic blood sugars," said Anna Tang Norton, who nursed for three or four months until her supply diminished. "I spent the first few weeks battling with many lows. Take advantage of the breast-feeding coaches at the hospital, ask many questions, and kick visitors out of your room so you can focus on breast-feeding. Call the help hotline once you get home."

- "Get either a Boppy or a My Brest Friend [both are nursing pillows]," said Shawna Trupiano, who is breast-feeding her 6-month-old. "Positioning of the baby [while nursing] is important, not only to get the most out every [nursing session], but to avoid improper latch techniques and possible pain from a c-section recovery as well."

- "It does get easier the longer you do it," said Joy McCarren, who nursed for 14 months. "They don't nurse forever, so if you have your heart set on nursing, remember that it is only for a short time, but the benefits and rewards are worth all of the struggles."

Formula Feeding

Maybe breast-feeding doesn't appeal to you or you need an alternative way to feed your baby. Welcome to the world of infant formula.

If you interview a potential pediatrician before your baby is born, ask him or her to recommend a formula. Of course, sometimes your child needs to weigh in before a formula decision makes sense. If your baby isn't tolerating a particular brand or version of formula, the pediatrician will let you know whether a change could help.

Research over the past 20 or so years has found a potential link between consuming intact foreign protein in early infancy (typically found in cow's milk–based formulas) and developing type 1 diabetes, explained H.-Michael Dosch, MD, PhD, a pediatrics professor at the University of Toronto and the senior scientist at the Hospital for Sick Children in Toronto, Ontario, Canada. Although research into this link was conducted around the world, the studies were often small and based on retrospective interviews rather than direct observation. Animal studies, using diabetes-prone mice, have shown the connection; human studies, though challenging and lengthy, are the next step.

The Trial to Reduce Insulin-Dependent Diabetes Mellitus in the Genetically At Risk (TRIGR) was founded by a small group of researchers in Canada and Finland and soon expanded to become the largest diabetes prevention trial.[3] TRIGR is now in its ninth year and running on three continents. It is following newborns from families with a parent or sibling with type 1. The trial will end in 2017.

TRIGR is exploring whether, to what degree, and how delayed exposure to intact food proteins (such as regular formula or foods with cow's milk) can reduce the chances of developing type 1 diabetes later in life, said Dr. Dosch, a cofounder of TRIGR.

From the late 1980s, he performed many of the animal and human studies that led up to the trial. In a November 2009 phone interview, he said that the type of infant formula *does* make a difference in terms of preventing the development of type 1 diabetes. "After 10 years of follow-up, our TRIGR pilot study found clear and significant evidence that, in infants with type 1 diabetic relatives, extensively hydrolyzed formula prevents the emergence of autoimmunity," he said.

For type 1 moms wondering what kind of formula is best to feed their children, "I would say to go with the hydrolyzed formula," said Dr. Dosch. These formulas include Nutramigen, the brand that is being studied in TRIGR, and Alimentum, a comparable brand that has been studied in animal research. "Probably either one is fine, but only Nutramigen is being studied in humans," he said.

Infants with a genetic risk for type 1 "tend to have an immature intestine which catches up in development over the first three to six months of life," said Dr. Dosch. It's during this period that exposure to intact foreign proteins such as those found in regular (not hydrolyzed) infant formulas represents a risk for developing type 1 diabetes. When the babies are a bit older, their digestive systems are able to process intact foreign proteins such as cow's milk formula normally.

Dr. Dosch noted that evidence is mounting that vitamin D supplementation also helps reduce the risk of developing type 1. The above formulas are pretty well supplemented with both vitamin D and DHA (docosahexaenoic acid), an omega-3 fatty acid that promotes brain development, which Dr. Dosch also recommends.

For type 2 moms, there are "absolutely no data," said Dr. Dosch, that suggest the type of formula intake can prevent the development of type 2. However, he said, "one risk that has been observed is that these mothers tend to overfeed their babies—and that must be avoided. They should follow the recommended amounts and scheduling for infant feeding."

People use formula for different reasons, sometimes in addition to breast milk.

"In the first couple months, I had to supplement with some formula," said Joy McCarren. "I went with a soy-based product because the doctors were concerned that my daughter may have adverse reactions to milk-based ones. I was more comfortable with the soy-based ones because I had an unsubstantiated fear of giving her milk-based formula."

Others felt the connection between cow's milk protein and diabetes was too speculative at the time they needed to use formula. "We tried a few different formulas, including lactose-free and soy-based, because my baby had diarrhea after drinking milk-based formula," said Suzie Won. "I didn't think that the cow's milk causing diabetes hypothesis was conclusive, so we used milk-based lactose-free formula, though I mostly relied on nursing."

Some women say diabetes had no influence on their choice of formula; instead, their hospital, a pediatrician, or some other factor influenced the decision. "I have used some formula to supplement when I am not available," said Shawna Trupiano. "I chose the brand of formula based on how well it mixes with water. I also chose it [because of] how it appears in the powdered form. I didn't like how [another brand of formula] mixes or smells or looks in the powdered form."

Up All Night

Sleep deprivation is one of the defining experiences of new parenthood. With a newborn who needs nutrition every few hours and who has no idea of the difference between night and day, nocturnal child care just goes with the territory. Sharing nighttime tasks with a partner who can help feed the baby, change a diaper, and secure you extra snacks or glucose at 2 a.m. can ease the burden.

Everyone says "sleep when the baby sleeps," and it's a good suggestion if the sleepless nights are truly affecting how you function during the day. Instead, I used my son's naptime to do things for myself, such as go online and read e-mail, which made me feel more connected to what was going on beyond the newborn haze. "I wish I had spent more time napping while my baby slept, but that was the only time to get things done," said Suzie Won.

Being woken up to tend to your baby in the middle of the night, again and again, can affect your well-being, make you crave carbs, and send your blood sugars into strange territory. Do whatever you can to maintain your health and sanity to get through it, and know that this period will pass.

"I think the lack of sleep, nursing and pumping all played a part in my diabetes management after having my first child," said Rachel Richer, 37, type 1, of Framingham, Massachusetts. Her kids are 4 and 2. "I didn't realize how much all of these things would impact my blood sugars." If you're awake and tending to your child in the wee hours, consider it another chance to see what the diabetes is up to, particularly if you often go low while nursing or pumping.

Just as pregnancy involved a new way of living and thinking, so too does new parenthood, particularly the sleepless nights. "I think the sleep deprivation issues are common among all new parents, but hit diabetics harder because of all the other things you must keep track of, including carb counts, bolusing, and testing," said Abby Nagel. "In order not to go completely nuts, I switched off nighttime duty with my husband, who fed our daughter pumped breast milk and then formula if she was still hungry."

The Baby Blues and Postpartum Depression

With all the hormones swirling both during and after pregnancy, plus all the new responsibilities of keeping a newborn alive, healthy, and happy, it is no surprise that your moods can jump all over the place. You might find yourself blissfully happy one moment, whimpering five minutes later, and rend-your-clothes sobbing soon after. I would find myself tearing up at the kind sentiments our friends had written on new baby cards. One nurse's "good luck!" note, scrawled on the side of a package of lanolin ointment, made me bawl. Most of the time, I knew the tears were hormonal, but sometimes they seemed to have a life of their own. This period, known as the baby blues, can last anywhere from a few days to a week or two after giving birth.

The Difference Between the Baby Blues and Postpartum Depression

The baby blues should not last more than two weeks, said Mary Beth Bahren. "If it does, call your doctor. If your doctor thinks you sound like you are dealing with postpartum depression, he or she will refer you to a mental health professional."[4]

Baby Blues
The baby blues can include mood swings (from happiness to sadness to anxiety to anger), feeling overwhelmed, crying, a lack of concentration, and difficulty going to sleep.

Postpartum Depression
Postpartum depression can start out with the baby blues symptoms, but things get worse and last longer. Signs include major moodiness, such as persistent crying, irritability, anxiety, or anger; more sleep issues, such as insomnia, restlessness, or, conversely, major fatigue; not wanting to eat or have sex; lack of energy, motivation, or simply any joy about anything; unexplained weight loss or gain; persistent feelings of shame, guilt, worthlessness, or inadequacy; avoiding your family or friends; difficulty bonding with your baby; thoughts about hurting yourself or the baby, or feeling like life isn't worth living.

If the tears don't go away, or if things get worse instead of better, you may be dealing with postpartum depression. This is a diagnosable condition that can be treated with medication, support, and counseling. Depression and diabetes go hand in hand, and even if you weren't depressed before pregnancy, it is possible to develop postpartum depression.

A 2009 study found, for the first time, definitive evidence that diabetes, depression, and pregnancy are linked. Katy Backes Kozhimannil, PhD, MPA, a research fellow with Harvard Medical School and Harvard Pilgrim Health Care Institute and the study's lead author, found that among more than 11,000 women, those with any kind of diabetes were about twice as likely than women without diabetes to develop depression during or after pregnancy.[5] "Postpartum depression is a serious illness that may be difficult to recognize, but can be treated once it is identified," said Dr. Kozhimannil. "Counseling may be all that is needed for women with mild symptoms. For more severe symptoms, depression can be treated with medication (antidepressants) and psychotherapy. If a woman is pregnant or breast-feeding, she needs to talk with her health care provider. Research indicates that some antidepressants can safely be used during pregnancy or by mothers who are nursing."

Finding others to support you during this new stage in your life can be crucial. "We've had a number of significant challenges, and I've definitely had some bouts of 'dark times' during the experience," said Bethany Rose, whose daughter came home after three weeks of intermediate care at the hospital. "I felt like I should be able to have this close bond with her, when really I felt like I didn't even really know her. That was hard. I have had some bad dark days. I treated it by leaning on my husband, my family, and everyone who offered help and support. I can't say it's totally gone now, but the bad days are definitely fewer and farther between."

If the walls seem to be closing in, consider a change of scenery— however temporary. There were some early times when I'd look out my bedroom window, feeling shackled to the electric breast pump, and I'd envy the people driving by who had the luxury of leaving their houses that day. That soon changed, and within a short period I became confident enough to leave my house to go places, learned to pump in my car while my kid hung out in his car seat (the pump adapter that plugged into my car and a hands-free pumping bra seriously changed my perspective), and eased back into life outside the newborn bubble. Slowly I felt like myself again, and you likely will, too.

"I am not aware that I suffered from postpartum depression, but I had days when I felt overwhelmed and exhausted," said Suzie Won. "Getting out of the house at least once a day really helped, as did simplifying household chores such as using paper plates and ordering take out."

Sometimes medication is necessary. Just as insulin helps your body process food properly, antidepressants can help your brain process certain chemicals that help maintain a sense of well-being. These can be ongoing or temporary meds, depending on your situation.

"I had postpartum depression with my first two kids, but being on Prozac before, during, and after my third pregnancy kept the depression from getting worse," said Michelle Kowalski. "I was taking Prozac when I got pregnant and my OB and I had read that babies born to moms taking antidepressants were more likely to have complications after birth. So I weaned off the Prozac and was miserable. My OB and I decided that the potential for complications was less of a concern at that point that my mental health, so I started taking it again, and continued on it while I breast-fed."

Some women need medication for only a limited time. Anna Tang Norton dealt with almost nonstop crying, insomnia, sadness, and anxiety, as well as very low blood sugars, two weeks after delivering her child. "Then, one day, about two weeks later, it completely went away," she said. "Strange, huh? It returned, full force, at around seven months. At this time, I visited my doctor and was put on [the antidepressant and antianxiety drug] Lexapro, at the lowest dosage, and I immediately felt better. It definitely helped perk me up and I used it for about four months."

Donations to Science: Diabetes and Pregnancy Research Studies

Depending on how close you live to major medical centers, you may have the opportunity to take part in clinical trials or research studies, either during pregnancy or afterward. These studies can help researchers figure out different elements of diabetes, pregnancy, and early childhood to provide further medical knowledge about diabetes, prevention, and early or alternative medical treatment.

There are pros and cons to becoming a research subject.[6] According to ClinicalTrials.gov, a website maintained by the U.S. National Institutes of Health, getting involved in a well-designed and well-executed study helps you take charge of your health, learn about and take part in new research treatments, get top care at some of the best medical centers before such treatments are widely available, and forward scientific research.

The risks include unwanted, major, or even life-threatening side effects to the treatment, ineffective treatment, and eating up a lot of your time and attention with trips to the study site, more treatments, hospital stays, or complex dosage requirements.

You can find out about studies funded by the U.S. National Institutes of Health (typically called clinical trials), how they are designed, the terms used, eligibility guidelines, and contacts for more information at www.clinicaltrials.gov. Type as many specific terms into the site's search engine as you can ("type 1 diabetes Boston" will find different studies than "type 2 diabetes pregnancy Texas," for example).

Sharon and her daughter are taking part in a multiyear study measuring whether delayed exposure to certain foods and food proteins protects against type 1 diabetes. Sharon has taken part in numerous studies for diabetes research and has long been involved with research endeavors. She and her husband decided, after much discussion, to enroll their daughter in the study.

"We didn't look at the study as anything that would change the way we raised our child, or what our expectations would be for any potential diagnosis," she said. "It was more about getting slightly better and more relevant nutrition information, and hopefully getting one step closer to understanding what role nutrition may play in diagnosis."

Because the trial is ongoing, there aren't a lot of solid answers yet. "We know of some people who were not accepted into the trials as their child didn't show the genetic markers, only to have that child diagnosed a few years later," said Sharon. "While we know that the genetic markers that they test for can be an indicator for higher risk, we also know that there may be more markers yet undiscovered. Also, even a positive genetic link doesn't mean absolute diagnosis. For those reasons, we try to minimize risk with some of the things we've learned about through nutrition and personal history, but we don't expect to have a diagnosis in the future."

Her daughter's blood draws for the study, which would otherwise be unnecessary, have been the hardest part of participating, said Sharon. "Our trial required blood work at 3, 6, 9, 12, and 18 months, and then yearly draws from 2 years through 10 years of age. So far we've just explained that sometimes doctors need us to get blood drawn, and we sometimes get our own routine testing done at the same time. Probably in the next year or two we'll be ready to explain a bit about what our daughter is involved in, and maybe let her decide if she is willing to continue participating. Originally it was only until age 5, but now it's been extended to age 10. We are unsure if its something we should continue to decide for her or not."

Despite not knowing whether her child will develop diabetes, Sharon said the extra monitoring provides more information about her daughter's health. "The one direct benefit we receive is that we are given [our daughter's] A1c and glucose value each time, so if something was starting to develop, we may find out about it sooner," she said.

Taking part in clinical trials isn't the right choice for everyone. Clemma Muller urges people to consider what they will do with the information gleaned from participating, particularly if the news is troubling. Her first son was recruited for a study about potential causes of type 1 diabetes while Muller was still in the hospital after giving birth.

"My husband consented to the study, which was testing for a genetic susceptibility to type 1," she said. "Our baby 'qualified,' which means he has the marker, but the people running the study dropped us because we [eventually] moved out of town. It was a horrible experience. I was devastated to learn that he had the genetic susceptibility, and they left us with no support or resources for dealing with this unwanted knowledge. Based on that experience, I have not participated in any other studies. I would certainly advise anyone considering a study to think about how they will feel about things they might learn, and get assurance beforehand that there will be support available if they do receive upsetting information, even if they are not able to continue with the study."

Birth Control

In the crush of everything you do day to day, finding time for sex may be the last thing on your mind. Or maybe not—a small percentage of women who go to their obstetricians for a six-week postpartum follow-up are actually pregnant again. If that is not your immediate plan, talk to your doc about birth control before you give birth or immediately after and use it consistently if you don't want to get pregnant soon.[7] If you are exclusively breast-feeding on demand for your child, it's likely that you aren't ovulating and won't get your period until breast-feeding slows down, but talk to your doctor about the specifics. If you want contraception, there are several options, particularly if diabetes is your only health issue. Even if it isn't, there's always a way to prevent getting pregnant again, and simple abstinence from exhaustion isn't your only choice.

Methods of birth control include hormonal contraceptives, barrier methods such as condoms (for men and women), diaphragms, cervical caps and sponges, insertable choices such as an intrauterine device (IUD), and spermicides. If you and your partner are done making babies, there are sterilization procedures such as a vasectomy for a man and tubal ligation for a woman.

Hormonal choices typically work by secreting the hormones progesterone, and sometimes estrogen, into your body to help prevent ovulation, change the uterine lining, and/or thicken cervical mucous—all of which inhibit or stop pregnancy. The Pill and the Mini-Pill are, respectively, estrogen-plus-progestin (a synthetic form of progesterone) or progestin-only drugs taken by mouth. The Implanon is a matchstick-like rod that is inserted under your skin for three years; progestin in the rod helps to prevent conception.[8] The Depo-Provera shot contains progestin; it is injected into the arm and lasts for up to 12 weeks.[9] A NuvaRing device goes into the vagina and has both estrogen and progestin that leech into the body; you replace it every three weeks.[10] The Mirena IUD can be inserted into the uterus for up to five years and secretes progestin locally; the hormone does not get absorbed throughout the body.[11] "I have a strong bias toward IUDs for monogamous women because of high efficacy and because they are metabolically neutral," said Dr. Florence Brown. "They don't affect lipids, blood glucose, blood pressure or increase the risk of blood clots."

The only hormonal birth control option considered safe during breast-feeding is the progestin-only Mini-Pill. It is not considered harmful in breast milk and might even slightly increase your supply. Combination pills with both progestin and estrogen aren't recommended for nursing moms because the estrogen can deplete your milk supply. You may notice an effect on your blood sugars with any form of hormonal birth control.

Nonhormonal contraceptives typically don't affect breast milk or supply and won't affect glucose control. The more common options include condoms, the diaphragm, the ParaGard copper IUD, vaginal sponges, and spermicidal creams, jellies, or foams. Condoms for men are thin sheaths fitted over an erect penis to block semen from entering the vagina. Far less common are condoms for women; these line the vaginal walls and are kept in place by one ring attached to the cervix and another ring just outside the vaginal opening. A diaphragm is a dome that covers the cervix and is used with spermicide; it needs to be refitted after you've had a baby. The ParaGard IUD works without hormones and is placed into the uterus; the copper in the device makes the uterine environment unfriendly for fertilization.[12] The vaginal sponge is made of foam covered with spermicide; it is inserted into the vagina and can be kept in place for 24 hours. Spermicides kill sperm and come in suppository, foam, cream, jelly, and film forms; they are often used together with barrier methods such as condoms or a diaphragm.

The natural family planning or rhythm method relies on you and your partner to abstain when you know you are most fertile and likely to ovulate, according to the timing of your period. Breast-feeding can affect this system, though, as you can be fertile before your first period arrives after giving birth.

If you and your partner know for sure that you don't want any more children, sterilization offers permanent birth control. In a tubal ligation, the fallopian tubes are blocked, tied, or cut to prevent ovulation. A vasectomy severs or blocks the vas deferens, which prevents sperm from exiting the body.

Work with your doctor to make the best birth control choice, and do your own research to ensure you're getting up-to-date information. "There are many myths that are not true about diabetes and birth control," said Dr. Tamara Takoudes. "Make sure your advice from your doctor is true, and if you are unsatisfied, then ask for a referral to a family planning clinic. Breast-feeding mothers cannot use any form of birth control with estrogen, but diabetes (without hypertension) is not as limiting as many patients think."

So, which to pick?

- "I am on the Mini-Pill," said Elizabeth Edelman. "I talked over the options with my OB and was on the Pill before. [My doctor] said the hormones in the Pill will affect milk supply and breast-feeding, but the Mini-Pill doesn't have all the hormones the regular one does. I've been on it for about five months now and have had no issues so far."

- "I'm about to start on the Mini-Pill," said Bethany Rose. "I definitely want to be on a pill because, frankly, condoms suck. But because I'm breast-feeding, I can't be on the regular Pill. I have to admit, though, that I'm about nervous about the Mini-Pill being slightly less reliable than the regular Pill, plus you have to take it at exactly the same time every day, because I'm *really* not interested in getting pregnant again in the next little while. So we may end up using a backup method as well. We'll see."

- "We have always used contraceptive foam before pregnancy, and we are continuing to do so now," said Joy McCarren.

- "I have a Mirena IUD because I got sick of having my period every month," said Amy Eddy.

- "I am considering an IUD without hormones to avoid the increase in clotting risks associated with the Pill," said Katrine Whiteson. "After having type 1 for 25-plus years and getting HELLP [a condition that includes the breakdown of red blood cells, elevated liver enzymes, and low blood platelets, which help blood clot] at the end of my second pregnancy, I think I already have increases in cardiovascular health risks and I would like to avoid further risks."

- "There are patients who just want to use condoms because they just want to be back in the pregnancy clinic in a year and want to plan a pregnancy around that," said Mary Beth Bahren.

- "My birth control is the same as before pregnancy—condoms," said Nicole Ishikawa. "Not by choice, but I cannot afford anything else."

- "Early on we used condoms," said Sharon. "But we used the rhythm method later as we'd had trouble getting pregnant the first time, so we didn't expect we needed much protection and would have welcomed a pregnancy had one happened."

- "After baby number one, I tried an IUD; after baby number two, we have been relying on condoms," said Clemma Muller. "The IUD never quite *settled* for me, and honestly, with two small children my husband and I rarely get those happy opportunities. Condoms make the most sense for now. Ultimately, my husband will get a vasectomy."

- "We relied on condoms and were not always 100 percent careful about it," said Suzie Won. "At 38, with nephropathy, I didn't think my body could handle another pregnancy. I'm surprised doctors didn't give me the option of having a tubal ligation, given my pre-existing complications. Perhaps because my first pregnancy outcome was better than doctors expected, they were optimistic about future pregnancies. It's easy for new parents to overlook something as important as contraception, and among the fragmented care of having multiple doctors, it's really up to the patient to make it a priority."

- "I never went back on birth control after fertility treatments," said Abby Nagel. "If I got pregnant again, that would be fine."

- "After the birth of my first son, I chose nothing in the form of birth control. As the birth of my second son approached, my husband was supposed to go have a vasectomy," said Shawna Trupiano. "I still have yet to see that one! I did not have my tubes tied because I felt like I went through pregnancy and birth and he could give a small sacrifice. As far as birth control now after my second child, total and complete abstinence. No time or energy for sex!"

Exercising Postpartum

Whether you worked out religiously throughout your pregnancy, did what you could, or never even broke a sweat, starting or getting back into exercise now that your baby is here is a good idea. Regular exercise is good for your blood sugar control (when done together with blood sugar testing, insulin adjustments, and managed food intake). Exercise also can help you shed baby pounds, prevent weight gain, and help you feel better mentally and physically.

If you had a cesarean, you may be told to hold off on any strenuous exertion until six weeks after your procedure. This typically gives your body enough time to heal. With an uncomplicated vaginal birth, you may be able to start working out moderately within a week or two.

Many places offer fitness classes or programs especially for new moms, including groups that work out while pushing kids in strollers, boot camps that have you hustling while an on-site babysitter watches your nonmobile baby, and gyms with on-site playrooms and babysitting. Some community centers open their exercise rooms to moms at specific times, and you can ride an exercise bike or elliptical while your baby naps in a portable car seat next to your machine. Check to see what your neighborhood offers.

Figuring out the logistics of exercise with a little one can be a challenge. More than a year after my son was born, I trained for and completed two sprint triathlons as a way to shed baby weight (and also because it seemed like a ballsy thing to do). I signed up and stayed on top of twelve weeks of daily swim, bike, and jog workouts. The toughest thing for me wasn't finishing (I was very much a back-of-the-pack athlete) or racing ("Compete to complete" was my motto). The hard part was coordinating childcare for our then-1-year-old with my husband's schedule and occasionally hiring a babysitter when I couldn't rise early enough to work out before Dave and Ethan woke up. On top of that, I'd run or bike with a glam fanny pack strapped above my tush so that I could easily carry my meter, a juice box or LifeSavers, some money, and an ID. It was hard enough to make time to work out, check my sugar, time the exercise to ensure my insulin wasn't peaking, and make sure my kid was okay without me; there were times when I wished I didn't have to schlep all my diabetes stuff around while jogging or cycling.

If such workouts aren't your thing, that's fine. Any kind of movement, from stroller walks to chasing after your kid, counts.

"I started walking four days after surgery," said Nicole Ishikawa. "I was proud to be on my feet for 15 minutes at a stretch, then it became 30 minutes and longer. I felt better by being outside and slowly walking. I may not see a gym in the next few years, but running around on playgrounds, walking with a stroller, and baby-and-mom fitness classes are so much more fun." Remember to carry what you need to treat hypoglycemia, even if you are just hanging out with your child by the swings and slide. "Having a toddler running around everywhere impacts your sugars," said Lindsay Gopin. "I often go low after playing in the park with her."

Sometimes it is easier to cover the exercise with extra food, instead of reducing insulin doses or timing workouts around kids' schedules. "I go to the gym on the weekend while my older son naps and my husband watches our 4-month-old, as well as at night when the kids are asleep after I nurse my youngest," said Katrine Whiteson. "Rather than trying to time a basal rate with these other things, I bring juice boxes to cover the exercise." Exercise isn't only an outdoor sprint or a gym class, either. "Our son was born in October, so some months, it was difficult to spend time outside," said Anna Tang Norton. "I used to walk the mall every Friday for about three hours. We became very acquainted with the baby changing room at Macy's!"

Returning To Work—Or Not

What you will do for your career when you have a child can be a tough decision or an easy one. If you need the income or love your job, you might not think twice about going back to work. If finances are less of an issue or you always planned to be with your kid while he or she was still a baby, staying home might be the simple solution. If you're weighing whether it makes sense to keep working, diabetes may play a role.

If you stay home, will the lack of a regimented schedule mean that you maintain or ignore a routine of regularly testing and treating your blood sugars? Will being away from a coworker's desk filled with penny candy help you avoid temptation, or is it too easy to snack from your own fridge if you're home all day? Will the loss of your income and benefits (which may include health care coverage) affect your household's budget significantly? If so, will your coverage for insulin, blood strips, and other diabetes equipment be affected? Can you continue to work part time or from home to maintain some income and adult responsibility? Who will care for your child if you plan to work full or part time? Can you get work done at home if your infant is pre-mobile, loud, or still not sleeping through the night?

"I stayed home with my baby," said Joy McCarren. "I learned I no longer had a normal routine, which messed up my diabetes care somewhat. I couldn't always eat at the same times that I was used to, and it was often hard to remember to check my sugar when I was feeling high or low if the baby was crying and needed attention." Anna Tang Norton found that staying home at first helped her regulate her diabetes and routines, so she felt confident when she eventually returned to work part time. "I took my maternity leave for 12 weeks, then gave notice," she said. "I think staying home was helpful in continuing to care for my diabetes. It was easier without having to focus on getting up in the morning, getting dressed, going to work, and so on. My diabetes has remained in control for nearly two years after I delivered, even when I returned to work part time seven months after delivering. I think I was able to organize my life and that of my family to encompass a newborn, a home, and my diabetes."

If you return to work, juggling bosses, a commute, and coworkers along with your family life can be a challenge. "I am teaching and had to finish the semester before I could take the summer off," said Nicole Ishikawa. "I crawled back into the classroom a week after my emergency c-section. I had my mom to help at home, and if I could have managed it any other way, I would not have gone back to work."

Other women say working full time was tough but ultimately didn't affect their overall health. "I worked full time with a commute when I was pregnant with my second child," said Katrine Whiteson, who was caring for her first child, a toddler, at the same time. "It was much harder for me to get exercise, and to even have time to test and bolus carefully, when I was pregnant and watching out for my 1-year-old. I'm not sure that less time working would have helped, but even out of this more chaotic situation, my blood sugar was almost as carefully controlled as it was in my first pregnancy, and I had another healthy baby."

Some Final Tidbits

Life as a new parent is certainly about a lot more than handling your diabetes in between the milestones and the tasks. Sure, the diapers are endless, but watching your baby smile and laugh for the first time is a lot of fun. Once you have a handle on things, some of the initial tasks get easier, which prepares you for the next milestones.

Establishing regular habits and keeping track of both your own needs and your baby's will help life move more smoothly. If you're schlepping a diaper bag everywhere, try to refill it every day at the same time so that you always have what you need. Pack it with extra snacks and sources of glucose so that you can treat reactions and hunger on the go. Do the same for your glucose meter if you're running low on test strips or other supplies, and don't let the rest of your supplies (e.g., syringes, pump supplies, CGM supplies, insulin, other meds) get too low before you restock.

"Routine is a mother's friend," said Yehudit W. "If you can set up your diabetes to expect the same every day, with a little variation of course, it will be much easier to focus your energy on taking care of the little one."

When your energy does flag, ask your partner, family, or friends for help, or look into hiring someone who can watch your child, even if you're home, so that you can get a break. While the idea of leaving your baby with someone else, particularly someone you don't already know, can be daunting, seeking out recommendations from friends, websites such as Sittercity.com, or companies in your area that screen and hire childcare professionals can ease your concerns. I'd fretted about leaving Ethan with a babysitter who wasn't family early on, but I managed to find a few caregivers I trusted. The first time I hired someone to watch my child while I worked in a different part of our house (on an early version of this book), it was phenomenal. I felt like an independent adult again for the first time in months, and my son had a great time playing with someone new.

"Take advantage of all the help you can get," said Anna Tang Norton, who was home alone with her infant son when a friend came to visit. "She asked if there was anything she could do. I asked her to just sit on the couch, watch TV, and listen for the baby, because I needed to lie down for just 20 minutes. It was the greatest gift. I also took advantage of help so I could change out my pump infusion sets, eat something to make sure my blood sugar didn't drop too low, and even so I could lock myself in my room to pump breast milk."

Flexibility and accepting that things won't run as smoothly as they used to, at least for a while, can go a long way in getting things done and moving through the day. I'm a big fan of to-do lists, and when I was up pumping in the middle of the night, I'd write down everything I hoped to accomplish in the short term. What I had been able to do in a day became a week's list of tasks once my son was in tow, and what I could once do in a week now took a month. I was also habitually late to things (Mommy-and-Me classes, meeting someone for a meal, doctor's appointments). Leaving the house with a baby was never a quick or simple process: it often involved a diaper change (or two), sometimes an outfit change, restocking and carrying the diaper bag and sometimes the breast pump, packing fresh bottles, and so on. I had to start getting ready to go somewhere a lot earlier than I ever had before. Plus, our house was often cluttered, which I learned to tolerate.

"You won't have control over many aspects of how things go," said Katrine Whiteson. "Somehow, you have to get comfortable with expecting the unexpected. This is definitely a big part of being a parent."

At some point, you and your partner might think about trying for another child. For some, thinking about the efforts it took to maintain tight control while pregnant keeps them from pursuing pregnancy again. Others can't wait to give their child siblings. If you're among the latter group, try to do all you can to get your blood sugars back into the recommended pre-pregnancy range.

"Plan ahead for the next baby," said Dr. Tamara Takoudes. "Many women will get pregnant and not realize that the hemoglobin A1c is crucial to having another healthy baby. It's important to be vigilant." Talk to your doctor about blood sugar recommendations and whether you should wait for your uterus to heal if you've had a cesarean, and see your obstetrician and endocrinologist for another preconception visit. Medical advice may have evolved since the last time you were there.

Good Luck With Everything!

So, here you are. Congratulations, Mama! Mazel Tov on your fantastic new baby! You made it through all the blood sugar tests, intense food scrutiny, glucose highs and lows, and who knows how many prenatal appointments and tests. Good luck as you venture into the brave new world of mothering with diabetes. After the rigors of pregnancy have receded in your memory, you may think that you're up for the challenge again, or you may decide that one pregnancy with pre-existing diabetes was more than enough for you. No matter what the future holds for you and your family, may you continue to be as healthy in parenthood as you were in pregnancy—and may we all continue to successfully manage our own sweetness within.

When Blood Sugar Control Isn't Enough

Appendix
Infertility and Pregnancy Loss

Your blood sugars? Great! Sex with your partner? Ongoing! Pregnant? *Sigh* . . . not yet. Dealing with infertility and diabetes can feel like an energy-draining double whammy of health issues. Not only are you constantly figuring out what to do to keep your blood sugars tight, but you're also probably watching the calendar to figure out when you're most fertile—and paying for and peeing on ovulation predictor kits to confirm this. Or maybe you're taking your basal temperatures every morning and watching the goop in your underwear to see whether you really are ovulating, and then—oh right!—you're hopping into bed with your partner to try, try, try to make a baby, already. This chapter covers what to do and whom to consult when nature isn't taking its course.

Most important, know that you're not alone.

Many of us require even more maintenance and medical specialists to figure out why, once again, our bodies aren't doing what everyone else's body seems to do naturally. For some women, getting pregnant isn't the problem—it's staying that way. Pregnancy loss is common even among women without diabetes. It is linked to higher A1cs, but if your sugars were in range and it doesn't appear that anything specific triggered a loss, the reason you miscarried might remain a mystery. The premature end of a wanted and possibly hard-fought-for pregnancy can be devastating. Yet it's definitely something you can learn to move past, as you cope with the loss and look forward to trying again.

What's Going On?

Infertility is an inability to get pregnant.[1] You are considered infertile after a year of actively trying to conceive (i.e., having unprotected sex around ovulation time) if you are younger than 35 or after six months if you're 35 or older, or if you have a history of many miscarriages. The time frame is key: it can take some fertile couples that long to conceive naturally, while older women are advised to seek help sooner because fertility declines rapidly with age. About 10 to 15 percent of all couples experience infertility, according to the MayoClinic.com.[2] Of those cases, about 40 to 50 percent are caused by female infertility, and another 30 to 40 percent are caused by male infertility. The rest are either a combination of male and female factors or simply unexplained—just one of life's many mysteries.

Several things can cause or lead to infertility, according to the U.S. national infertility association RESOLVE: age, weight, sexually transmitted diseases (STDs), fallopian tube disease, endometriosis, exposure to the chemical diethylstilbestrol (DES), smoking, and alcohol use.[3] As a woman, your fertility declines the older you get—starting around age 27, but dramatically dropping in your mid- to late thirties, and becoming the exception rather than the rule once you hit your forties. Men aren't exempt from this, either. A 2003 study found that men in their late forties took five times as long to get their partners pregnant than men in their twenties.[4]

For women, being significantly obese or underweight also can affect fertility. Any STDs you or your partner acquired long before trying to conceive might cause problems or affect your partner's sperm, and some STDs may have no other symptoms beyond conception problems. Fallopian disorders include blocked or scarred tubes as a result of prior STDs, earlier pelvic surgery, or a history of abortion. Endometriosis, where uterine tissue is found outside the uterus, which can cause painful and heavy periods, has also been linked to infertility. So has being exposed to chemicals or toxins such as those you ingest if you smoke or drink alcohol. You might also face problems if your mother, while pregnant with you, took DES, a hormone that was given to some pregnant women through the early 1970s to help with pregnancy bleeding and miscarriage.

Diabetes and Infertility: Are They Related?

While all the above are general causes of infertility, what's going on when you have diabetes? According to Dr. Carol Levy, type 1 or type 2 may have an indirect role. "Poor glucose control may create an environment where someone might not get pregnant because the body doesn't view the environment as appropriate for becoming pregnant," she said. Because conception requires specific timing, eggs being released, sperm being hardy, and your body being hospitable to nurturing for the next 40 or so weeks, if something in your chemistry isn't exactly right, you may have a tougher time procreating.

Then again, despite the potential risks, plenty of women with high A1cs get pregnant, so blood sugars aren't the only factor when it comes to figuring out why you're not yet knocked up. Type 1 women, who develop diabetes because of the body's autoimmune response, are prone to developing other disorders such as thyroid disease or autoimmune premature ovarian failure. The body might decide to wrongly attack healthy cells that maintain thyroid hormones or ovarian function—both of which play a role in getting pregnant. Talk to your doctor about checking your thyroid levels and ovarian function, particularly your levels of TSH (thyroid-stimulating hormone) and FSH (follicle-stimulating hormone). Your TSH level should be checked before you try to conceive, but definitely look into your TSH and FSH levels if you're trying and not succeeding.

Another below-the-belt issue is polycystic ovarian syndrome (PCOS) or having polycystic ovaries. This is common in type 2 women and appears in some type 1s. With PCOS, the follicles on the ovaries, which typically release eggs when you ovulate, instead form cysts or lumps. These cysts don't break open, the eggs are trapped inside, and ovulation doesn't happen. Without ovulation, there's no egg to fertilize. Coupled with irregular or missing periods, PCOS puts a serious damper on your efforts to conceive. The condition can be treated with medication that enhances ovulation, such as Clomid or drugs that make you more sensitive to insulin, as insulin resistance often goes hand in hand with PCOS.

Extra pounds can affect your efforts to get pregnant, too. "Type 2 diabetes has a higher association with obesity, and obesity has an association with sub- or infertility as it affects ovarian function," said Dr. Tamara Takoudes. "For example, when obese women lose weight, they ovulate more predictably."

Losing weight helped Brandie Poole, 28, type 1, PCOS, of Summerville, Georgia. She is now 15 months pregnant after trying for 1½ years. "My reproductive endocrinologist advised me to go on a restricted diet in order to help me with the insulin resistance and lose weight. I lost 35 pounds," she said. "Also, having type 1 diabetes and polycystic ovarian syndrome is demanding. I have to strictly watch what I eat in order to lower my insulin needs. If I don't lower my insulin, I am less likely to ovulate."

Sometimes, though, diabetes has nothing to do with why you aren't getting pregnant. "Our infertility has been unexplained—every test came back normal," said Melissa Baland Lee, 30, type 1, of Allen, Texas. She tried to conceive for eight months and is now six months pregnant. "That was the oddest thing to hear as a type 1. I'm not used to hearing that there's not a problem!"

Beyond fooling around for fertility's sake and having nothing to show for it, what can you do to get past the problem?

The Infertility Workup

The ins and outs of the infertility world are vast, and while this book gives an overview of what's available, other books, websites, and blogs get more specific (see Resources). Many procedures, known as assisted reproductive technology (ART), and medications can help you get pregnant. For some people, financial, religious, or personal reasons put some elements of fertility treatment beyond reach, although there are ways to tackle fertility within religious parameters and financial plans can help offset (but rarely relieve entirely) the often staggering costs of treatment. For other people, including myself, the possibilities that exist with ART are truly phenomenal and are the only way to get and stay pregnant and ultimately experience what it is like to have children with a genetic and biological link.

If you are having trouble conceiving, talk to your gynecologist or endocrinologist about getting referred to a reproductive endocrinologist, who will check you and your partner out. Your regular gynecologist may prescribe clomiphene citrate (Clomid) to help you ovulate, and that could be all you need. However, after close to six months of Clomid alone, talk to a specialist who understands infertility's intricacies and will do all the appropriate testing to try to figure out the root of the problem. It doesn't make sense to pop a pill to help you ovulate if your partner's sperm has problems, for example, and you wouldn't know that without the right diagnostic tests. So don't dither if your own doc isn't moving forward with a referral to a fertility specialist, particularly if you've been at this for several months and doing the work to keep your sugars tight.

"Some doctors will suggest you get the workup after three or four months of trying to conceive, because you're trying so hard to keep your blood glucose control in range," said Dr. Levy. Figuring out the problem will take time. Your doc will likely give you a diagnostic exam that includes an analysis of your and your partner's full health history, a vaginal exam, a Pap smear, several blood tests, a sperm analysis, a history of your menstrual cycle and any irregularities, and possibly one or more invasive tests to determine whether your uterus, fallopian tubes, and ovaries are fully functioning.

The fertility workup is intense, but it can uncover any number of issues that might be preventing you from getting pregnant and carrying a baby to term. Ovulation problems can be tweaked with drugs such as Clomid to help your eggs to be all they can be. Other oral meds include metformin (Glucophage), which helps women with insulin resistance. If you have PCOS, metformin can help even out your periods and induce ovulation.

Progesterone is prescribed to help the uterus maintain a pregnancy-friendly environment and can be taken alone (by mouth, as a suppository, or as an intramuscular injection) or as part of an in vitro fertilization (IVF) cycle.

Your doc may also prescribe baby aspirin, which makes the blood thinner and less likely to clot. This helps with some health issues and can aid embryo implantation.

Other meds are used to control or manipulate the monthly cycle. They can be prescribed on their own or as part of ART. Some drugs prevent your body from producing normal hormones before your period arrives. Others stimulate the ovaries to produce follicles that contain eggs. Still other meds help trigger ovulation so that an assisted conception can take place at your most fertile time.

Intrauterine insemination (IUI) is when fresh or thawed frozen sperm is inserted directly into your uterus using a catheter. Some IUI devices are medicated to enhance your chance of conception and pregnancy; others do not use additional drugs. In either case, the egg and sperm hopefully fertilize inside your body. Two weeks after ovulation, a blood test determines whether you are pregnant.

With IVF, you take medication about a week before your period to suppress the beginnings of your next cycle. Once you begin your period, you inject a drug to stimulate your ovarian follicles and cut back on the suppression med. At the same time, your follicles are typically monitored regularly via vaginal ultrasound and blood work— perhaps every other day or every day—and the amount of stimulant drug is watched to make sure the follicles grow at a good rate. When they've reached the right size, the stimulant drugs stop. You then take a trigger shot to induce ovulation. Shortly thereafter, your eggs are retrieved from the follicles in a procedure that typically involves light anesthesia and are fertilized with your partner's sperm to become embryos. A few days later, depending on how many have fertilized and thrived, one or more embryos are transferred back into your uterus via a catheter. Less than two weeks later, a blood test confirms whether you are pregnant.

If too many follicles grow, you risk developing ovarian hyperstimulation syndrome (OHSS), which can halt or slow an IVF cycle. OHSS happens when there is too much fluid in the ovaries, which can affect other parts of the body, and it requires immediate treatment. It can be particularly tough to handle while managing diabetes. Alison, 30, type 1, of England, has been trying to conceive for four years. She used Clomid alone and did one IVF cycle and one in vitro maturation cycle. In vitro maturation is similar to IVF but does not use follicle-stimulating drugs; it is used for people with polycystic ovaries. Alison experienced OHSS in her first IVF cycle, and it was rough: "Constant vomiting made my diabetes tough to control, and I had ketones," she said.

With diabetes already on your plate, the idea of fertility treatments might make you worry about carrying more than one child at a time (or "high-order multiples"). With IVF, it's common to want to transfer more than one good-looking embryo to increase the possibility of having at least one develop into a healthy pregnancy. Relax—if you approach ART responsibly, you will not become the next Octomom. While Clomid and IUIs can increase your chance of having multiples, working closely with your fertility doc and your endocrinologist should help determine exactly what those chances are, as well as how your diabetes (and eyes, kidneys, or other body parts) might be affected. A multiple pregnancy (twins or higher) with diabetes also seriously increases your chances of developing pre-eclampsia, which can mean an earlier or premature delivery. Your docs will talk to you about newborn health problems that are more common with premature births.

Your fertility doctor might discuss other IVF-related procedures with you if they are recommended with your health history. These include third-party reproduction, in which donor sperm, eggs, or embryos can be used to help you conceive and carry a pregnancy.

When Fertility Drugs and Diabetes Intersect

Different drugs affect people in various ways. With any medication, your reproductive endocrinologist might not know how your blood sugar control will react. "Fertility doctors were often unable to answer even basic questions about whether the drugs tended to increase or decrease insulin requirements," Alison said. Clomid "caused a huge rise in insulin requirements around five days before my period, much greater than I'd experienced before. I ended up increasing my basal rates by about 75 percent and doubling my insulin-to-carb ratios. I found the progesterone I had to take caused a large increase in insulin requirements—around 20 to 40 percent more. My blood sugars were erratic prior to the embryo transfer, then settled down."

She dealt with the changes by tweaking her insulin doses and checking her sugars often. "Having a CGM and insulin pump made a real difference to my control," she said. "I could see constantly what was happening to my glucose levels and take action quickly."

If you're on multiple daily injections, keep a close eye on how you might need to adjust your doses. Lisa used metformin and Clomid for four months and is now 25 weeks pregnant. "I didn't have any changes while taking Clomid. I found, post-ovulation, I needed more insulin than pre-ovulation. I tested and corrected more often, and also regularly took long-acting insulin at 3 a.m. in addition to my normal morning and bedtime doses of long-acting."

Other meds, particularly progesterone, can affect your blood sugars. Christi Tipton tried to conceive for seven years and did several medicated IUIs, then stopped when she learned of the impending arrival of her adopted daughter, now 3. Tipton conceived a second daughter, now three months, without treatment. "Taking progesterone orally, versus suppositories or injections, always made my blood sugars rise," she said. "I was not given any specific instructions on how to handle those, since I had such good control over my blood sugar anyway that I felt the occasional higher (but not too high) numbers at the time were not detrimental."

Other drugs can require insulin adjustments. "I had to run a slightly higher basal rate when on birth control pills, which was the first thing I went back on at the beginning of my cycle," said Kathryn, who had twins after IVF. (Birth control pills are sometimes prescribed as part of IVF to help regulate your menstrual cycle.) She found she needed a correction bolus for the injection that triggered ovulation, as well as more insulin for progesterone shots. While she was under anesthesia for the egg retrieval, she said, her sugars dropped slightly.

"The drugs I took were very typical for an IVF cycle, and I maintained an A1c in the sixes throughout my cycle," she said. "I don't know how I would have been able to make the corrections I needed in order to maintain great control if I had still been on multiple daily injections of insulin."

Other women don't notice so many changes. "I was lucky in that none of the drugs I used for IVF seemed to cause problems with my blood sugars," said Carol Speight. She did one round of IVF after trying to conceive for a year, and her daughter is 5. "I maintained very tight control prior to the procedure. I wasn't really that stressed when going through IVF, which is strange, I know. We were very lucky and I got pregnant on my first attempt. I don't know if this attitude would have been different if it had been our third or fourth."

Dealing with infertility on its own is a huge juggle of doctor's appointments, invasive and potentially uncomfortable tests, blood draws, figuring out what insurance will cover and how to pay for what it will not, timing and waiting, and ultimately determining how much treatment you want to pursue (and whether the options of donor sperm, donor eggs, surrogacy, adoption, or choosing to live childfree are considerations for you and your partner). Throw the rigors of diabetes into the mix, and you may wonder what you ever thought about before these health issues were a part of your life.

Before I got pregnant with our son, Dave and I tried to conceive for several months on our own. We then met with a reproductive endo as soon as we could. Many diagnostic tests, a few months of Clomid, three IUIs, and an IVF cycle later, our son was conceived. The whole process took a year. At the time, I worked in an open-plan office, so I had a lot of hushed cell phone conversations with assorted nurses and doctors, who would wait on hold while I rushed into the one conference room with a locking door. Other times, I simply left the office, grabbing a pen and paper, and stood outside talking furtively on the phone while trying to write down exactly the advice or results I was hearing. I then would go online and read countless websites and blogs to decipher what I was supposed to be doing at what time of the month. (Waiting for ovulation? Counting down to have bloods drawn on day three of my cycle? Ordering medication that wasn't covered by my insurance and trying to do it as cheaply as possible? Signing up for additional insurance coverage? Scheduling a follow-up doctor's appointment?) We were one of those "unexplained infertility" couples, though my age probably played a role. Regardless, juggling infertility along with type 1 took up a lot of mental energy.

Stress Effects

Infertility equals stress. Whether or not there's an explanation for why you can't get pregnant, you're still doing a lot of waiting for the right time of the month and subjecting yourself to tests, insurance questions, financial issues, and feelings of disappointment, sadness, and anger—all while trying to keep those sugars tight. It ain't easy. Your blood glucose numbers can be affected, even if you are being super-vigilant about everything you eat, the insulin you take, and the exercise you do (or aren't doing, if your doc has told you to stop or lighten up on the workouts to enhance fertility).

"The stress of infertility made my blood sugars unpredictable," said Laura, 39, type 1, of New York City, who did six IUIs and one IVF cycle and is now 20 weeks pregnant with twins. "Worry, anxiety, hormones, depression, fatigue, multiple appointments, financial worries, and food cravings are undoubtedly the ingredients for the proverbial recipe for disaster. It's frustrating and overwhelming. I broke down a few times because I'd bolus normally for a meal, [only] to find my blood glucose was 350 mg/dL two hours later. In those moments, I'd feel like, 'Well, there it is, Laura, you ruined *everything*. You don't deserve to be a mother. You have no self control and you just *suck*.'"

These are pretty powerful drugs you're on, and they can do crazy things to both your sugars and your state of mind. It's hard to tell yourself that it is not your fault. For now, it just *is*. Try to be kind to yourself; bolus or inject some insulin, drink some water to flush out any ketones, go online to find some kindred spirits, and do whatever you can to get past it. Treat the highs as soon as possible, and trust that you're doing all you can to keep you and your potential baby as healthy as possible.

It took a year for Sharon to conceive her first child, now 4, and she has just started trying to conceive her second. She did two unmedicated IUIs after spending several months doing the initial infertility workup. "I think it affected me in that every month when we weren't pregnant, after having tried so hard and done so well at good control, it felt like a slap in the face," she said. "Most months, I spun out of control during the other two weeks. Eventually, it raised my A1c to 7.8. I was actually told the month we conceived [when her blood was drawn at the same time for both a pregnancy result and an A1c], that we'd have to stop trying to conceive until my A1c was under control."

Dealing with two health issues that require so much attention makes it hard to chill out about either of them. "The stress was incredible," said Randi Schwartz Carr. She tried for two years and conceived her daughter through IUI; she also had four miscarriages. "Part of the stress I felt was put on myself. I felt like my body couldn't do anything right: type 1 diabetes and then I couldn't stay pregnant. Even thinking about going through the whole process again puts me in a frenzy."

Your state of mind can affect what's going on, as well. "Stress makes my blood sugar shoot up to the 300s or more," said Tanya Duncan, 31, type 1 of Seattle, Washington. She has tried to conceive for five years using Clomid, "obsessive charting of my blood sugars," and timing, as her husband is in the military and isn't always home when she is ovulating. "If I start thinking about how much I want to be pregnant, or how grown up my baby would be if I had gotten pregnant at X (my age, a particular event or holiday), my blood sugar hits 350 mg/dL easily. If it's just the low-level stress of temping [taking early morning temperatures, which shift higher when ovulation is imminent], waiting for a positive result on an ovulation prediction kit, and then the inevitable disappointment, my blood sugar is in the mellow 200s. Essentially, the only time my blood sugar is good is after the crushing arrival of Aunt Flo [my period]."

Despite her history, Duncan and her husband were successful. She is now five months pregnant.

Stress relief differs from person to person, but learning to manage it can only help. "I don't think the stress has affected my diabetes any more than other stress," said Alison. "I do feel extra pressure to make sure my diabetes is very well controlled. I need to know that I'm doing everything I can to make sure my diabetes doesn't impact the chances of the treatment working."

Relying on your loved ones can help, too. "Infertility is a hard road to take, and you must have the complete support of your partner or spouse when you are going through it," said Abby Nagel. It took six months and a medicated IUI for her to conceive her older daughter, now 6, and three IUIs and two IVFs over six months to try to conceive her second. (She ultimately conceived her younger daughter without treatment.) "I cannot stress how important it is to have a partner to talk things out with and to help. You cannot do all of it alone. Between the shots, daily appointments, awkward testing, and procedures, it is not easy. Be prepared and be tough—that is the only way to handle the bad news as well as the good news. Keep positive thoughts, because when it works, it is unbelievable."

Food for the Best and Worst of Times

Eating throws another curve ball into the diabetes and infertility game, and it can split the month you are trying to conceive into two distinct blocks. The first is the two-week stretch just after you've ovulated, or done an IUI, or done the embryo transfer procedure of an IVF or frozen embryo transfer cycle. You could be pregnant (or, with some fertility treatments, you are pregnant until proven otherwise). This was a time when I drank skim milk and seltzer instead of Diet Coke, snacked on carrots instead of crackers, and worried about whether my apples were organic and my salmon was wild or commercially farmed. I became extremely conscientious about what I ate because of what could be—before actually knowing whether I was actually pregnant. Eating so healthfully was much easier on blood sugars, helped me believe my potential embryo was thriving, and made me think much more about what I put into my mouth. However, it was a lot more effort and thought, and frankly it was not much fun. I had far more insulin reactions, which I treated judiciously with small sips of 100-percent juice or something else equally healthy. I also thought longingly about the deli meats I once ate, the blue cheese that used to flavor my salads, and the preservative-filled ice cream and snacks I really enjoyed. I also learned what it's like to feel pretty close to having an insulin reaction all the time, though my hypoglycemia unawareness was and remains pretty strong. (I can easily feel normal but be hanging out in the 50–60 mg/dL range. As a reminder, though, you should not try to drive a car, care for other children, or do much at that lower range without treating to go slightly higher to a healthy range of 70–99 mg/dL.) I never drank as many juice boxes as I did when I thought I might be—or was—pregnant. I tried to think of them not only as blood sugar treatment but also as fruit servings for a fetus.

Then there are the next two weeks of the month, after finding out pregnancy didn't happen. I thought of this, quite simply, as a food freefall. I ate whatever I wanted because I could—and covered with giant insulin boluses of insulin. Sure, my sugars soared, but they came back down to a normal range. Eventually. This was also a quick way to pack on extra weight. None of it was particularly healthy in the long term. But in the short term, it was one way to help feel better after the disappointment of a negative pregnancy test.

Such patterns are common when dealing with the roller coaster of fertility treatments, blood sugar control, and the finality of a negative pregnancy test:

- "I ate really healthy during the time I was ovulating to the time AF [Aunt Flo, my period] arrived," said Tanya Duncan. "And then I fell apart and ate salt-and-vinegar potato chips twice a day for a week."

- "I really try to eat as though I am pregnant so that I can keep my blood sugars in a good range," said Heidi, who has tried for a year to conceive her second child. "You can't do that indefinitely, though."

- "I had more times I felt 'diabetes burnout,' where I felt like I put all the extra effort into controlling my blood glucose for nothing," said Lisa, who tried to conceive for 15 months and did four rounds of Clomid. "As time went on my discipline and motivation for blood sugar control decreased." Her efforts paid off, though: Lisa is now 25 weeks pregnant.

- "I tend to eat less healthily than I should, so the changes I was making for the potential life inside of me should have been the way I ate in general," said Sharon. "Without that extra motivation, I would drift back to my less-healthy habits. Also, people didn't know I was trying to conceive, and switching my habits and mulling over them to think about if I should or shouldn't have a particular fish, or a drink, or a sugar substitute, can call attention to your TTC [trying to conceive] journey—which was unwanted."

- "When things fail and go to hell, I plow through chocolate— more I think than I would [if I were not] affected by infertility," said Carlynn. She has stopped trying conceive after six years and two miscarriages. "Infertility and pregnancy loss steer me toward chocolate like nothing else."

And Yet More Doctor Appointments

Meeting with an infertility doc and eventually going through treatment means entering into a whole new round of physician visits, timing, blood tests, procedures, and so on. It's like being diagnosed with a chronic illness again: novel words, new docs, unfamiliar procedures, and more. How much time all these new appointments will take, particularly if you end up doing one or more IVF cycles, might, once again, become something to consider if you work in an office. (See Chapter 4 on how to handle time away from work.) These meetings can eat up your allotted time off, or even your livelihood itself. "I am a teacher and am only given a certain number of days off per year," said Brandie Poole. "The fertility specialist is over two hours away from where I live. When we went, my husband and I both had to take a full day off from work. It wasn't much of a problem for me because I had some days saved up, but if I ran out of days, I would not get paid for them. My husband [an insurance agent] has to make up the days he took off on the weekends." Melissa Baland Lee had a similar tale: "Scheduling doctor's appointments around work is always difficult. I am a contractor and lost at least $600 of work because of appointments that had to happen on specific days in [one] month."

Others do what they need to do and are lucky to work in an office where it's not a problem. "I do take more than my fair share of time off from work to take care of my health," said Tanya Duncan, whose endocrinologist's office is an hour away and whose OB/GYN, who prescribed Clomid and monitored progress via ultrasounds, required a lot of visits. "Working from home is not an option. But my office is supportive, so it hasn't been an issue."

Telling others that you are dealing with infertility has its pros and cons. If you and your partner want to keep things to yourselves, people won't ask you for updates ("What did the doctor say?" "Was the IUI successful?" "Are you pregnant yet?"). This can be a relief. However, staying mum can make people wonder what's happening if they see you leaving for appointments without explaining why.

"I was lucky—I work in a family business," said Randi Schwartz Carr. "What was not great was that I didn't share our troubles with my family. I was constantly going for testing or to other appointments. My family thought something was seriously wrong with me. I know they assumed it was my diabetes. I usually would say that I was going to the endocrinologist. I just didn't say which one, and they didn't know to ask. I also tried to schedule things for early in the morning."

Some clinics have early morning appointments (from, say, 6:30 to 9:30 a.m.) so that you can schedule blood tests or ultrasounds before work hours. Other clinics rely on the patient to get in early to get out early. At the practice where she did her IUIs and IVF, "the way it worked is that monitoring appointments are first come, first served between 7 and 8:30 a.m.," said Laura. "I made a habit of arriving by 6:45, and got on the subway at 6:15 to make it. You sign in and then wait. At 7, the staff arrives. Generally, they'd call me in for a blood test by 7:15, and I'd be seen between 7:45 and 8 for the 15 minutes it took for the ultrasound, measuring and counting follicles, and the adjustment to the medication regimen. Then I'd run out the door to take another train for 45 minutes, just to get to work by 9. No one at work was the wiser. But if I arrived later, signing in tenth or eleventh instead of fifth or sixth in line, which happened occasionally due to train delays, it could make me very late, and I'd be extremely anxious."

Some people need to take time off during the workday or leave early to get to the clinic before it closes for the evening. "I tried to schedule appointments around lunch time or at the end of the day to limit the disruption to my normal working schedule," said Carlynn. "I learned to keep the rest of my life as free from engagements as possible."

The medication regimen for ART can be complex. Fertility medications may need to be injected or taken at exactly the right time, similar to taking insulin before meals or reducing insulin basal rates before exercise. Christi Tipton needed to take intramuscular shots for her IUIs and relied on her husband for help. "The hardest part was planning and doing injectables at a time that worked well for my and my husband's schedule," she said. "He helped me give some shots in my behind—it was hard to reach. We had to plan the first several shots to be done at my work because my schedule was changing and we needed them to be at the same time every day. Work, while we didn't tell them it was fertility related, did accommodate and allowed me to use a 'health room,' which had a chair, a couch, and a bathroom. So he would come to my work and give me the injections at the same time every night until my schedule changed shortly thereafter. It was a challenge, but doable."

Other women tell their employers what is happening and say it makes things easier when leaving the office for appointments. "I was very open," said Amy Eddy. She tried to conceive for three years and did three IUI cycles before getting pregnant without treatment. "I definitely had to take time off, mostly because the fertility clinics are out of the area. It wasn't a problem for my job because my boss and coworkers were understanding." Abby Nagel had a similar situation: "I scheduled appointments so I could go to them before I went to work," she said. "I had a good working relationship with my immediate boss, so she was aware of what I was doing and worked with me so I could do my job and attend the doctor's appointments I needed to go to."

Final Words of Infertility Wisdom

Sometimes, the best advice comes from the women who have walked the walk before you. I learned that I needed to screen any calls with pregnancy test results. If you are waiting for a nurse to call you with the results of your lab pregnancy test, consider whether you want to hear the news in person or in a voicemail. At first, I eagerly answered my cell phone when Caller ID showed my clinic was calling. But I could tell right away if the result was negative—just from the tone of the nurse's voice—and I always wanted to hang up when I heard it. I learned to let the call go straight to voicemail and gave my clinic permission to leave the results there (be sure your clinic knows it's okay to leave messages for you; some are reluctant to do so if they think someone else might hear the information). That way, I could process the test result myself without needing to talk to anyone until I was ready. Plus, if you're lucky enough to hear it, it's nice to listen to the voicemail that says you are pregnant, again and again.

Here is what other women who have faced similar struggles learned:

- "Talk to your endocrinologist about your struggle," said Melissa Baland Lee. "My endocrinologist was my guide in my quest to conceive, as she had been so active in my efforts to reach my A1c goals for the years leading up to that point. She counseled me, dictated a time frame on how long to try before consulting a specialist, and then gave me a recommendation for a fertility doctor she trusted who had worked with her diabetic patients."

- "Infertility's tough," said Carlynn. "It's very tough and most of your friends will not have much useful information. Some will blame it on the diabetes; have information and data to correct that belief, either just for yourself or for anyone who you want to correct. Others, however, can offer tremendous support as they will be there to listen and take your mind off the topic for a few hours."

- "If possible, it's important to pick a fertility practice that is supportive rather than just pushes you through the process to an end goal," said Sharon. "I felt we were being pushed to try too many new things at once." She said her clinic encouraged her to use medications, but she and her husband instead implemented several lifestyle changes and chose to do two unmedicated IUIs, one of which was successful. "I'm so glad I trusted my gut and did not try so many things at once," she said.

- "Write down everything that you put in your mouth, and the time and date," said Abby Nagel. "That was a huge help in figuring out how to maintain some control over hormones, insulin, and what my numbers were."

- "Infertility is frustrating, especially if you are not given a reason for it," said Joy McCarren. She tried to conceive her first child for six years and has been trying for several months for a second. "Trust your body. If you feel something is wrong, push your doctors to keep checking. Even if all the tests come back normal, it can still take months or years to successfully conceive. However long it takes, do not let infertility become the main focus of your life. Focus on the positive things, and avoid being around people who make you uncomfortable because of their attitudes, or [because] they are pregnant, or seem to get pregnant by just thinking about it."

- "It's terrible and I wish it on nobody," said Amy Eddy. "I think it changed me a little. I did not want to be inadvertently insensitive to others who may experience it and ask stupid questions and make stupid comments. I had other friends who dealt with infertility for years, and once they had their kids, it was like they totally forgot what it was like when speaking to me, who was still childless and depressed. I promised myself I would never forget what it was like."

- "Set realistic goals with what you can do to go through the treatments and the regimen for taking fertility shots in addition to managing your diabetes in a healthy way," said Abby Nagel. "Find a way to balance all the things you need to do."

- "The thing about infertility and having type 1 for me is that I feel like I expect things to go wrong, and when they do, I feel like I just need to keep moving forward," said Randi Schwartz Carr. "I don't let much hold me back."

- "It's so easy to get caught up in the cycle of disappointment each month if you don't get pregnant, and to take progressively worse care of yourself, diabetes and otherwise," said Sharon. "Find some balance that will allow you to keep positive and to remember that it is just as important to take care of yourself whether you are pregnant this month or not."

It may be hard to fathom if you're in the midst of it, but you can eventually move past infertility. Knowing all the options when dealing with infertility can help you learn which step is best to take for you and your partner when planning to build or grow your family. Dealing with infertility and diabetes needn't define you. Instead, work with your doctors, within the parameters of these conditions, to figure out what needs to be done so you can get to where you want to be: a healthy mom with a healthy baby.

Pregnancy Loss

Maybe you got pregnant easily, or maybe it took a lot of effort. It may be early in your pregnancy, somewhere in the middle, or at term. No matter your history, learning that a pregnancy has ended before it should have can be a disappointing, painful, and sad experience.

Miscarriage, also called spontaneous abortion or pregnancy loss, is common.[5] It's believed that between 10 and 20 percent of all pregnancies end in miscarriage, with some estimates reaching higher, as many pregnancies end so early that a woman might not even realize she was pregnant (and might think she was just having a particularly heavy and slightly late period). On the other hand, you may be in a doctor's office having an ultrasound when you learn, without any warning, that the pregnancy has ended. Pregnancy loss can occur anywhere from the earliest stage through full term, and it comes with its own vocabulary. A *blighted ovum* describes a pregnancy in which the embryo didn't develop properly or stopped growing early. A *chemical pregnancy* is another early loss; it occurs after you've gotten a positive pregnancy result but before a gestational sac or fetal heartbeat can be seen (typically, around week five or six). Miscarriage that happens before the end of the twelfth week, roughly the first trimester, is called an *early pregnancy loss*. A *clinical miscarriage* occurs anytime after a gestational sac and heartbeat have been seen. A *missed miscarriage* happens before week 20 and is discovered when there is no fetal heartbeat or fetal growth, which indicates fetal death, but there are no other signs or symptoms of miscarriage and the fetus is not passed from the uterus on its own. A pregnancy that ends after the twentieth week is called a *late-term loss* or *stillbirth*.

If you are reading this section and are worried about or have experienced miscarriage, I am sorry. (And if you are reading this chapter but weren't worried about miscarriage, this does not mean that a miscarriage will ultimately happen to you.) Such a loss does not preclude you from carrying another pregnancy to term and having a healthy baby. Signs of a possible miscarriage include vaginal bleeding (brown, pink, or red), abdominal cramps, and the lack of pregnancy signs you felt before, such as breast sensitivity or food and scent sensitivities (although feelings of nausea and fatigue normally subside around weeks 10 to 12 of pregnancy). Even with these symptoms, though, the pregnancy may be fine. Always contact your doctor if you notice these issues.

A doctor will confirm a miscarriage after a pelvic exam and an ultrasound that shows the pregnancy has not progressed to where it should be based on the date of your last period. If you are still in the early weeks of pregnancy, blood tests that measure the levels of hCG, a hormone that's evident only when you are pregnant, will be done to confirm whether the levels are increasing properly. (They typically double every few days.) If the numbers are rising but not at the right rate, you may have an ectopic pregnancy, which is a pregnancy that's developing in the fallopian tube instead of the uterus. This is a serious issue, as the tube could burst and might need to be removed if the pregnancy continues. Otherwise, if you are past the first five or six weeks, your doctor can do a vaginal ultrasound to see how big the fetus is and whether it has a heartbeat.

If you have miscarried, your doctor will give you options. It is possible to wait and have your body pass the fetal tissue on its own, though this can take some time and cause major anguish; your doctor may ask you to collect the tissue for testing. Another option is to do a D&C (dilation and curettage) or D&E (dilation and evacuation), where the fetal tissue is taken from the uterus by scraping or vacuum. This is typically done under a light anesthesia, and the tissue is tested to try to determine what happened.

If you have more than two or three losses, you are considered someone with recurrent miscarriage. This warrants a trip to an infertility or high-risk specialist. Other books and resources go into more detail about miscarriage, including specifics about potential causes. For any woman, these can include chromosomal defects, infections, high fevers, hormonal imbalances, autoimmune problems (in addition to diabetes), anatomical abnormalities in the uterus or cervix, and blood incompatibilities or immunological problems where the body attacks the cells of the embryo or the placenta.

Was It My Fault? Was It the Diabetes?

In many cases, if your A1c is within the recommended preconception range, diabetes likely did not cause the miscarriage. "It is hyperglycemia that causes spontaneous abortion/miscarriage, not diabetes per se," said Dr. Lois Jovanovič. "If blood glucose levels are high during conception and thereafter, the embryo does not form correctly and there is an increased rate of a blighted ovum. If the blood glucose levels are normal at the time of conception, there is no increased risk." Dr. Tamara Takoudes concurred: "Type 1 and type 2 diabetes increases the risk of miscarriage, especially with poor or less-than-optimal glycemic control, due to unknown causes," she said. "The best remedy for this is diligent and compulsive control prior to conception. Once conception has happened, better control is good, but the horse is out of the barn already."

Other factors include PCOS or a history of missed or erratic periods. "Because diabetics are more likely to have irregular cycles, the ovulatory cycles they do have may be less fertile, have lower hormone levels, and may not adequately support pregnancy," said Nanette Santoro, MD, professor and director, Division of Reproductive Endocrinology and Infertility at the Albert Einstein College of Medicine and Montefiore Medical Center, and president of the Society of Reproductive Endocrinology and Infertility. "Also, women with PCOS, for reasons unknown, have a consistently higher rate of miscarriage than the general population."

There are also vascular concerns, noted Dr. Carol Levy. "People with type 1 or type 2 may not have adequate placental flow, and this can affect blood circulation," she said. "That's why you get the close fetal monitoring [later in pregnancy] to have a sense if something is going on. Nonstress tests are a very indirect measure of how the placenta is functioning. If the baby's heart rate doesn't increase a specific amount for a specific duration of time, there might be a problem with the placenta." Because it's unknown whether tight glucose control eliminates the potential for problems related to vascular disease, women with low A1c tests still get extensive fetal monitoring, Dr. Levy said.

Coping With Miscarriage

Once you've been through the physical experience of pregnancy loss, the emotional realization kicks in. It's hard not to question what you could have done differently.

"Try not to fixate on blaming yourself," said Ani Collum, 32, type 1, of South Boston, Massachusetts. She had one miscarriage just before she was diagnosed with type 1 diabetes and is now seven months pregnant. "After my miscarriage, I found myself rehashing every moment of my pregnancy in my head to see if I could pinpoint the cause. Did I exercise too hard? Did I push myself too much at work and let the stress get to me? Did I not eat enough well-balanced meals? Did I miss any signs of diabetes prior to the miscarriage? I thought about these things constantly."

Collum's story is unusual in that her diabetes diagnosis came at nearly the same time as her miscarriage. However, her feelings are common to women experiencing nearly any type of pregnancy loss.

"Miscarriage is rough for anybody that has to go through it," said Brandie Poole, who has had two miscarriages. "Don't make it harder on yourself by blaming it on something you could or could not have done. Sometimes we ask *Why me*? And there may not be a reason why. Have faith. Just because you miscarry doesn't mean you won't ever get pregnant again."

It's your decision whether to tell others what you have gone through, how much to mourn the loss (whether privately or with others), and when to begin focusing on the future. I learned while writing this book that an early pregnancy had evolved into a missed miscarriage. The embryo never developed at the rate it should (the hCG test results were always below normal and never doubled) and stopped developing entirely around week five. In week seven, I had a D&E. Dave wondered why I seemed to get over it so soon, but I was frankly so used to having things not progress properly with my health history that I felt it didn't make sense to feel bad about it for even a short time. I was more impatient about getting past this particular pregnancy effort and just wanted to move forward.

For others, a miscarriage hits hard. Sarah Savage prepared herself for pregnancy by going off the Pill and taking daily prenatal vitamins, fish oil, folic acid, and calcium, and she got the go-ahead from her internist, OB/GYN, endocrinologist, ophthalmologist, and dentist to try to conceive. She also cut out all alcohol, tested her blood sugar 12 to 14 times a day, ate only organic and all-natural foods, increased her intake of protein, and made sure to eat low-mercury fish when she ate seafood at all. Finally, her husband took over all kitty-litter changing responsibilities (cats' fecal matter can carry toxoplasmosis, an infection that can harm a fetus). They bought a chemical-free wool, cotton, and natural latex mattress, and she saw an acupuncturist to help prepare her body to adjust to going off the Pill and to enhance fertility. She also tracked her basal temperatures and cervical fluid to determine when she was most fertile.

She got pregnant the first month she and her husband tried to conceive.

"We were thrilled and a bit shocked it happened so quickly—and four pregnancy tests confirmed it," said Savage, 30, type 1, of Santa Barbara, California. "We were so relieved my diabetes hadn't affected our ability to get pregnant. We told our immediate families right away, because our parents have been hoping for their first grandchild for years. At six weeks, I started spotting and completely freaked out."

Savage called her OB/GYN's office and spoke with a nurse who told her many women spot during pregnancy and are fine. However, Savage continued to bleed and went to her doctor's office for a blood test.

The test came back with my hCG level at 54, and I was devastated to learn that at six weeks, it should have been 1,000.

I redid the blood test again a few days later (it was 56) and again a few days later (it was 32). The doctor confirmed that this meant I was having a miscarriage. They weren't sure why I lost the pregnancy, but they said it either didn't implant properly in my uterus, or the cells didn't divide properly and my body knew something was wrong and let it miscarry.

After the miscarriage was confirmed, I just broke down and cried. I was on the verge of tears for about a month. My husband was very sad, but stayed strong for me. He picked up a lot of the chores and responsibilities for me so that I wouldn't have to think about them, which was very kind and helpful. At the time, I didn't think I was depressed, but looking back, I see that I was. I was eating differently without knowing it, and couldn't get up the energy to go to the gym, yet somehow I lost five pounds. After it was confirmed, I still didn't believe it entirely until we told our families. That's when it really felt real. I felt a sudden gush of reality when I called my dad and recounted all what had happened, then repeated everything for my mom. They were very supportive and reassuring about it all.

Before Savage conceived, two friends had told her about their own miscarriages, and she knew they had gone on to have healthy babies. "Knowing about these experiences made me feel so much better when it happened to me," she said. "I didn't feel alone."

She decided to share her story via e-mail to her friends. "Writing it out made me feel better," she said. "I think it really helped my emotional recovery process to share. If a miscarriage happened to any of my girlfriends, I didn't want them to feel alone. This way, even if they never told me about it, they would know that they weren't alone."

In response, Savage got a barrage of e-mails and phone messages offering support. "At first, I couldn't answer any of them because I wasn't ready to actually talk about it," she said. "It's a lot easier to type it than say it out loud. It took me a month before I could actually respond, but just reading and hearing their kind words helped me so much."

Savage continued acupuncture to help her get through her depression and to recover physically from the loss, and she waited for two periods (on her doctor's advice) before gearing up to try to conceive again. "My doctors say we're good to go, so we're starting this month.

I'm a bit more wary this time around, and probably won't share the next pregnancy with family until we're further along. But I'm feeling recovered, emotionally and physically, even though I get sad when I think about it. I know it sounds cliché, but I know that baby wasn't meant to be. I'm not sure why, but it's better that it happened when it did, rather than later in the pregnancy. Fingers crossed, all goes well."

Where Miscarriage and Diabetes Meet

Whether it's the stress of learning what is happening, different hormones, or something else, diabetes control can be problematic during a miscarriage, particularly if you were on medications such as progesterone during the pregnancy. Randi Schwartz Carr, who had four miscarriages before conceiving her daughter, now 2½, noticed this. "My hormones were always wonky," she said. "It became extremely hard to control my diabetes, especially since I would get pregnant and then miscarry."

Others notice that their blood sugars calm down after a miscarriage. "I had a positive pregnancy test, and at that point my insulin requirements were up about 30 percent, but the levels were stable," said Alison. "I miscarried at six weeks. At that point my insulin requirements dropped rapidly—returning to normal levels after about five days."

Some people say that a miscarriage does not affect blood sugar numbers at all. Such tight control at least lets you know that diabetes probably didn't cause the loss. "Tight control reduces all these risks of miscarriage, stillbirth, and other medical conditions that could increase infertility," said Dr. Tamara Takoudes. "That being said, no assumption can be made that there is no risk, as the general risk of miscarriage can be as high as 20 percent, and the risk of birth defects in the general population is 2 to 4 percent. Ferreting out the effects of medical disease is very hard with such high baseline risks. Tight glycemic control is optimal, though, in reducing the risks."

Pregnancy Loss: Advice From the People

Your doctor will likely offer you sincere condolences for what happened and may refer you to resources for dealing with loss. But sometimes the best insights come from others who have suffered similarly:

- "Be your own advocate," said Brandie Poole. "If you want answers as to why you miscarried, ask for them. Don't let the doctor blame it on your diabetes, especially if you know your diabetes has been under control."

- "What is so irritating to me is that many doctors associate every little thing you have to your diabetes," said Randi Schwartz Carr. "I wish someone in our struggle would have been more willing to step outside the box and help us. We were lucky to find that in our reproductive endocrinologist. It doesn't just have to do with fertility—it has to do with all the aspects of a person with diabetes. It infuriates me that if you have diabetes, you can't have a simple hangnail; its root has to be the diabetes."

- "Know you're not alone," said Sarah Savage. "Allow yourself to grieve. Cry. If you're not okay, show it. Talk about it if you can. Write about it—journaling can be very cathartic. Talk to your doctor and bring your husband with you to keep him involved in the process. The more he's involved, the more he can support you."

- "Everyone deals with miscarriage in their own fashion," said Carlynn. "I needed time and space to be alone. My sister offered to make a scrapbook of my pregnancy, and it was the last thing I wanted. Listen to yourself and do what you need."

- "Be prepared for some very out-of-range blood sugars," said Joy McCarren, who had one loss at five and a half weeks. "My sugars went very high during my miscarriage. I'm guessing due to stress, and my A1c actually went up over half a point. You have to let yourself grieve and recognize that, no matter how far along you were, you've lost a child. That will bring with it all the normal stages of grieving. Don't be surprised if you begin to feel upset again as your due date approaches. Even if you've been feeling totally fine about the miscarriage for months, it can still affect you as the day draws closer to when your baby would have been born."

- "I've learned the hard way that people mean well, but almost never have anything really good to say about it," said Christi Tipton, who has had four miscarriages. "They often end up saying things that make you feel a lot worse. Ignore all well-meaning family members and friends who think they have great advice but really don't. Grief comes in all shapes and sizes, and the grief I felt with each miscarriage was different than what others may experience in a lot of ways. But you need to experience it and give yourself permission to be okay again, because it is the only thing that will allow you to move on, emotionally."

- "I was shocked by how much I cried," said Alison. "I literally couldn't stop crying for several days after the miscarriage, and I started to think it might never stop. When I look back, it's easy to see that a lot of that was caused by hormones, and I improved rapidly as my hCG levels dropped. I think time is the most important thing. We went away on holiday pretty soon afterwards, as we felt we needed to get away from our busy lives, and just have time to come to terms with it and move on."

- "Know it happens for a reason," said Heidi, who has had two miscarriages. "Something was wrong. Just continue to exercise and watch your sugars so you can try again."

- "Two things really helped me, and they were great distractions," said Sarah Savage. "First, a friend sent me the *Twilight* book collection, and I read all four books in three weeks. Every night they provided me a great escape. Second, there was a fire here in my town and we were evacuated. It was four horrible days of not knowing if we'd lose our house, but it was four days of not crying all day. Our house was fine, but this fire helped me to adjust my priorities a bit. The miscarriage had happened, and I couldn't do a damn thing about it. The fire forced me to let it go a bit and focus on my own survival."

No matter how you choose to handle the medical and emotional issues that come with pregnancy loss, know that miscarriage or stillbirth doesn't mean that parenthood is permanently out of reach. Do what you can to get past the loss—or losses—until you feel you're ready to try again. Loss is an unfortunate detour, but it's not a dead-end. With time, medical help, and whatever else you may need to help complete your family, it's possible to reach your goal of having a thriving baby and being a mom—who just happens to have diabetes.

Glossary

Albumin: proteins that, when secreted in the urine, can be a sign of early kidney damage.

Amniocentesis: A test that measures a sample of amniotic fluid for potential genetic problems. This test can also confirm if a baby's lungs are fully mature if a premature delivery is necessary.

Basal rate: The minimum amount of insulin required to keep your blood sugar level while you are not eating. An insulin pump delivers a basal rate 24 hours a day.

Biophysical profile: Fetal monitoring tests that measure breathing, moving and muscle tone while in utero. Typically done with nonstress tests.

Blood sugar: The amount of glucose in the blood, measured in the United States as milligrams per deciliter (mg/dL).

Bolus: A dose of insulin taken via an insulin pump generally before a meal or to correct a high blood sugar (correction bolus).

Carbohydrates: Also called carbs or carb. Food measured in grams of carbohydrate are most likely to affect blood sugar levels. Carbohydrates includes foods such as breads, grains, pastas, fruits, some vegetables, and other starchy or sugary items.

Certified diabetes educator: a health care professional who is trained and certified in diabetes and who works with patients to help learn how to better manage the condition.

Cesarean section (c-section, cesarean delivery): An operation that involves opening the abdomen and uterus surgically to deliver a baby.

Chorionic villus sampling: A test that analyzes the tissue of the placenta and can determine if the fetus has genetic disorders.

Continuous glucose monitor (CGM): A device attached to the body that continuously reads your blood sugar levels. A wire inserted under the skin monitors blood sugar fluctuations. A CGM is typically used with an insulin pump and a handheld blood glucose monitor.

Correction factor: how many points a blood sugar reading will drop when taking one unit of insulin. A correction factor of 1:50 means one unit of rapid-acting insulin will drop a person's blood sugar by 50 points. Used to treat high blood sugar readings.

Creatinine: a kidney waste product that accumulates in the blood when the kidneys are malfunctioning.

Dawn phenomenon: The morning blood sugar rise that happens when your body sends out hormones as you prepare to wake up. Setting a higher basal rate upon waking or eating more protein as a bedtime snack can help counteract this increase.

Diabetic ketoacidosis: when very high levels of blood glucose, combined with too little insulin, cause the body to develop ketones. Can lead to coma and death if not treated immediately.

Doula: a person who supports a woman before, during and after childbirth.

Endocrinologist: a doctor who specializes in disease of the endocrine system, such as diabetes.

Epidural: Anesthesia injected through a tiny plastic tube into the epidural space, which is just outside the membrane covering the spinal fluid in the lower back. It offers pain relief during labor and/or delivery.

Estrogen: a hormone produced by the ovaries.

Fetal echocardiogram: a test that analyzes fetal heart development.

Fingerstick: A way to obtain a drop of blood from the fingertip to test blood sugar levels.

Folic acid, folate: a B vitamin that helps prevent neural-tube defects when taken in adequate amounts before and during pregnancy. Folic acid is the synthetic form of folate, which is found in foods such as orange juice, legumes and leafy green vegetables.

Glucose tablets: Tablets of pure sugar, sold in most drugstores. Less tasty than most candy. They're a way to get measured amounts of glucose into you when treating an insulin reaction or hypoglycemia.

Group B strep: a bacteria found in the vagina that can require antibiotics during labor so that a newborn isn't infected while passing through the birth canal.

Hemoglobin A1c: The average of your last two to three months of blood sugar readings, which shows how much glucose you have spilled over that time. Nondiabetic numbers are 4 to 6 percent, while people with diabetes are encouraged to maintain A1cs at 7 percent or lower.

Hyperglycemia: High blood sugar.

Hypoglycemia: Low blood sugar. *See* insulin reaction.

Hypoglycemia unawareness: When you don't feel the symptoms of an insulin reaction or low blood sugar or until it is much lower than where you typically feel them.

Inducing labor: If you don't go into labor naturally, a doctor can, using medication or other methods, cause you to start having contractions.

Infusion set: The tiny plastic tube that's inserted under the skin and transfers insulin from an insulin pump to the body.

Insulin: a hormone that regulates blood sugars and converts food into energy.

Insulin pump: A device, which looks like a beeper or cell phone, that automatically delivers insulin to a person with insulin-dependent diabetes. Can be worn on a waistband or tucked into a bra; some models can be worn wirelessly. It delivers both basal (ongoing) insulin and bolus (for meals) insulin. Works together with an infusion set.

Insulin reaction: A term for a low blood sugar reading or hypoglycemia, typically 59 mg/dL or lower during pregnancy and 79 mg/dL or lower pre- or post-pregnancy. Also known as low blood sugars or lows. Symptoms typically include feeling sweaty, jittery, drained, or unable to think clearly or slurring speech.

Insulin resistance: When the body needs more insulin than is normal to process glucose in the tissues and prevent the breakdown of fat. Insulin resistance is normal in pregnancy, and it increases as pregnancy progresses as a result of the hormones produced in the placenta.

Ketones: When blood sugar levels are high, fat instead of glucose is broken down for energy. When this happens, ketones spill into the urine from the blood. Their presence is a sign that blood sugar levels need to come down immediately. They can also be a sign that your body is using ketones for energy if you aren't eating enough calories.

Lancet: A small, sharp device used to help puncture the skin to produce a drop of blood.

Lochia: The blood and bits of uterine lining that leave the uterus after giving birth.

Maternal-fetal medicine specialist: a doctor who specializes in high risk pregnancy.

Midwife: a person trained to assist women in childbirth; provides a more holistic approach than an obstetrician/gynecologist typically would.

Multiple marker tests: Screenings done during pregnancy that indicate whether the fetus is developing as expected. These include blood tests and ultrasounds such as the nuchal translucency test.

Neonatal intensive care unit (NICU): A unit in the hospital that has special equipment and trained staff to care for premature or seriously ill newborns.

Nonstress tests: Monitoring that measures fetal heart rate and movement as well as placental function.

Nuchal translucency test: an ultrasound that measures the space in the back of a fetus' neck and can determine the risk of some chromosomal abnormalities.

Obstetrician/gynecologist: Also known as an OB/GYN. An obstetrician is a doctor who delivers babies while a gynecologist is a doctor who specializes in women's health, particularly the female reproductive system.

Ophthalmologist: an eye doctor.

Perinatologist: a doctor who focuses on the care of the fetus during a high-risk pregnancy.

Placenta: develops alongside a fetus in the uterus. It serves to nourish the fetus and eliminate fetal waste products.

Postprandial blood sugar: The level of blood sugar after a meal or snack.

Pre-eclampsia: a serious condition that develops during pregnancy that includes high blood pressure and fluid retention. Requires immediate medical care.

Progesterone/Progestin: Progesterone is a hormone that supports pregnancy and is involved in the menstrual cycle. Progestin is a synthetic form of progesterone and is used in birth control pills.

Rebound high: When blood sugars go really low, typically overnight while you are sleeping, the body releases hormones that help raise the sugars quickly so that your brain can still function. Also called the Somogyi effect.

Retinopathy: damage to the retina, the thin lining in the back of the eye. High blood sugars can damage the blood vessels in the retina.

Spinal: Anesthesia delivered through an injection into the spinal fluid that gives pain relief during labor and/or delivery.

Ultrasounds: The use of ultrasonic waves to examine the uterus and monitor a fetus during pregnancy.

Vaginal delivery: Delivery through the birth canal and the vagina.

Resources

Diabetes/Pregnancy Websites and Online Communities

Diabetic Mommy

Bulletin boards and other resources about all forms of diabetes, pregnancy, parenting, and trying to conceive.
www.diabeticmommy.com

TuDiabetes

A community of people touched by diabetes, with several active boards devoted to pregnancy and diabetes.
www.tudiabetes.org

Diabetes Forums Pregnancy Threads

Separate areas for pregnancy with type 1 and pregnancy with type 2 diabetes, among other subcategories.
www.diabetesforums.com/forum/diabetes-and-pregnancy/

Diabetes Blogs

The Diabetes OC (Online Community)

An umbrella site for the hundreds of blogs devoted to living with diabetes. Blogs are broken down into type 1 and type 2 bloggers, as well as by other categories, and you can find bloggers writing specifically about pregnancy, either currently or in the past.
www.thediabetesoc.com

Managing the Sweetness Within

This is my blog, which chronicles my efforts to get and stay pregnant while living with type 1 diabetes; it is the precursor to this book. Come take a look if you've read all the way through to here and liked what you read!
www.thesweetnesswithin.blogspot.com

Diabetes and Pregnancy/Parenting Yahoo groups

To read and contribute to these groups, whose posts are delivered to your mailbox as individual e-mails or daily digests, log into groups.yahoo.com and search for the group you want to join.

Positive Diabetic Pregnancies

As of February 2010, a very active group.

Pregnant Pumpers

Less activity here, but the archives are worth checking out, and the group may be busier by the time you read this.

Diabeticmoms

Regular postings by those who have moved past pregnancy and are now balancing parenting with diabetes.

Diabetes in General

Books

Beaser, Richard S., with Amy P. Campbell. *The Joslin Guide to Diabetes: A Program for Managing Your Treatment.* Simon and Schuster, 2005.
    More detailed explanation of the condition from the topnotch medical center for diabetes.

Gehling, Eve. *The Family and Friends' Guide to Diabetes: Everything You Need to Know.* Wiley, 2000.
    What to hand to your loved ones if you don't want to explain it all yourself.

Jackson, Richard, and Amy Tenderich. *Know Your Numbers, Outlive Your Diabetes.* Da Capo, 2006.
    Written by a Joslin physician and the creator of the popular blog DiabetesMine.com.

Rubin, Alan L. *Diabetes for Dummies.* 3rd edition. Wiley, 2008.
    A good basic book that explains things as simply as possible.

Scheiner, Gary. *Think Like a Pancreas: A Practical Guide to Managing Diabetes With Insulin.* Da Capo, 2004.
    All about living with diabetes and being on insulin.

Websites/Online Communities

Diabetes Daily

A support network for people affected by diabetes, with forums, blogs, and recipes.
www.diabetesdaily.com

DiabetesSisters

Advocates for improving the health and well-being of women with diabetes.
www.diabetessisters.org

Diabetes Talkfest

A site to support young adults, adults, families and friends who have been affected by diabetes. Message boards and chat rooms.
www.diabetestalkfest.com/

DiabeticConnect

The world's largest online community for people living with diabetes.
www.diabeticconnect.com

Diabetic Rockstar

A social networking site focused on newly diagnosed, in-need, or uninsured people with diabetes.
www.diabeticrockstar.com

dLife

For your diabetes life—a website and television show that address daily diabetes management. Site includes blogs, recipes, articles, advice, and more.
www.dlife.com

Juvenation

A type 1 diabetes community created by the Juvenile Diabetes Research Foundation.
www.juvenation.org

The Diabetes Resource

A comprehensive directory covering every aspect of diabetes, including pregnancy as well as medical professionals, support groups, blogs, insurance resources, and more
www.thediabetesresource.com

Trying to Conceive

Book

Weschler, Toni. *Taking Charge of Your Fertility*. HarperCollins, 2002.
How to figure out when you are most fertile, using the fertility awareness method.

Nutrition/Carbohydrate Count in Foods

Book

Heller, Richard F., and Rachael F. Heller. *The Carbohydrate Addict's Gram Counter*. New American Library, 1993.
    Despite its misleading title, I have used this pocket-sized guide for years to figure out the carb counts of many meals.

Websites

Calorie King

Has a food search database to look up the carb counts in specific foods.
www.calorieking.com

USDA National Nutrient Database

Details of the nutrients and vitamins in food from the U.S. Department of Agriculture.
www.nal.usda.gov/fnic/foodcomp/search

Logs for Blood Sugars, Insulin, Food, and Exercise

Websites

Medtronic Daily Journal

I began downloading this page years ago and continue to use it to keep track of blood sugars and other information. These records can be easily faxed to a doctor's office, too.
www.minimed.ca/download/Documents/Daily%20Journal%20Log%20Book.pdf

SugarStats

A free and subscription-based website for online diabetes management. Allows you to enter and track your blood sugar readings to see trends.
www.sugarstats.com

General Pregnancy

Books

Murkoff, Heidi, with Sharon Mazel. *What to Expect When You're Expecting*. 4th edition. Workman, 2008.
    Considered the bible by many, and the best-selling pregnancy guide out there. Some feel it gives too much detail on what could go wrong during pregnancy, but I think it is comprehensive and straightforward.

Iovine, Vicki. *The Girlfriend's Guide to Pregnancy.* 2nd edition. Simon and
   Schuster, 2007.
   This is an insider's guide from one woman's, rather than a medical profes-
sional's, perspective.

Insulin Pumps/Continuous Glucose Monitors

Books

Kaplan-Mayer, Gabrielle. *Insulin Pump Therapy Demystified: An Essential
   Guide for Everyone Pumping Insulin.* Da Capo, 2002.
Walsh, John, and Ruth Robert. *Pumping Insulin: Everything You Need for
   Success on a Smart Insulin Pump.* 4th edition. Torrey Pines, 2006.

Website

Insulin Pumpers

Extensive site and forum about all things pumping and insulin pump–
related.
www.insulin-pumpers.org

Bed Rest

Websites

Pregnancy Bed Rest

Judith Maloni's site, featuring information and support for families and
caregivers.
fpb.cwru.edu/Bedrest

Sidelines

The national high-risk pregnancy support network. Offers telephone buddy
system and other resources for women on bed rest as well as women with
other pregnancy complications, including diabetes.
www.sidelines.org

Diabetes and Exercise

Book

Colberg, Sheri R. *Diabetic Athlete's Handbook.* Human Kinetics, 2009.
   While this only touches on pregnancy, it is a detailed look at exercise and
diabetes, whether you are a hardcore athlete or your workouts are more
recreational.

Website

Diabetes Exercise and Sports Association

A group that works to enhance the quality of life of people with diabetes through exercise and physical fitness.
www.diabetes-exercise.org

Birth Plans

Websites

PregnancyToday

Create your personal birth plan.
birthplan.com

BabyCenter

Another site to help you build a birth plan.
www.babycenter.com/100_create-your-own-birth-plan_5235284.bc

Birthing Naturally

How to write a birth plan.
www.birthingnaturally.net/birthplan/how.html

Diabetes and Parenting

Book

Palmer, Kathryn Gregorio. *When You're a Parent With Diabetes: A Real-Life Guide to Staying Healthy While Raising a Family.* HealthyLivingBooks, Hatherleigh, 2006.
A practical guide written by a long-time type 1 woman with two kids (and a type 1 husband). Great insight.

Breast-Feeding/Pumping

For more resources, talk to the lactation consultants at the hospital where you deliver, and/or ask your baby's pediatrician for referrals to lactation consultants.

Book

Huggins, Kathleen. *The Nursing Mother's Companion.* 5th edition. Harvard Common Press, 2005.
One of the more comprehensive books on the topic.

Websites

Attachment Parenting International

A parenting style that stresses a close, highly responsive relationship between parent and child. Regardless of how you feel about the philosophy, the site's forums on breast-feeding can be helpful for advice and support. **www.attachmentparenting.org**

KellyMom

Covers breast-feeding, along with other parenting topics such as sleeping.
www.kellymom.com/bf/index.html (for general information)
www.kellymom.com/bf/concerns/mom/diabetes-maternal.html (for advice specific to moms with diabetes)

La Leche League International

All about breast-feeding. Offers support, encouragement, information, and education.
www.llli.org (for general information)
www.llli.org/cbi/bibdiabetes.html (for a selected bibliography on breast-feeding and diabetes)

MOBI Motherhood International

Mothers Overcoming Breastfeeding Issues. Support and information for when breast-feeding doesn't come easy.
www.mobimotherhood.org/MM/default.aspx

Ask Moxie

A blogger and mother who posts about why nursing is so hard, with info for moms with PCOS.
moxie.blogs.com/askmoxie/2006/01/breastfeeding_w.html
Part 2: "What's the normal learning curve?"
moxie.blogs.com/askmoxie/2006/01/breastfeeding_w_1.html

Yahoo Group

PumpMoms

Very active group offering tips on pumping breast milk, exclusive pumping info, and advice on related issues.

Research Studies

Websites

Clinical Trials

To volunteer/qualify for a medical study on diabetes (and/or pregnancy).
www.clinicaltrials.gov

Type 1 DiabetesTrialNet

A worldwide network of researchers studying how to prevent, delay, or reverse type 1 diabetes. Provides information on screening and clinical trials for type 1.
www.diabetestrialnet.org/index.htm

Infertility/Pregnancy Loss

Books

Aronson, Diane, and the staff of RESOLVE. *Resolving Infertility.* HarperCollins, 1999.
An informative and straightforward guide.

Ford, Melissa. *Navigating the Land of IF: Understanding Infertility and Exploring Your Options.* Seal Press, 2009.
Written by a blogger whose site is the go-to place for infertility. The book contains insight from more than 1,500 blog readers. It is compassionate, understanding, and even laugh-out-loud funny in parts.

Vargo, Julie, and Maureen Regan. *A Few Good Eggs: Two Chicks Dish on Overcoming the Insanity of Infertility.* Regan Books, 2005.
Two women who have dealt with infertility offer insight and advice.

Websites/Online Communities

RESOLVE

The National Infertility Association. Provides support groups, information, and opportunities to meet and connect with others dealing with infertility.
www.resolve.org

IVF Connections

Share advice and ask questions of others dealing with infertility on these infertility bulletin boards.
www.ivfconnections.com

Cyclesista

A monthly list of bloggers who are undergoing infertility treatment. Want to find others who are dealing with IUI, IVF, or frozen embryo transfer at the same time as you? Here they are.
www.cyclesista.com

Blogs

Stirrup Queens Blogroll

A compilation of more than 1,800 blogs about infertility. Diabetes blogs, including mine, are listed under "Situation Room/More on the Plate: IF and Health Issues."
www.stirrup-queens.com/a-whole-lot-of-blogging-brought-to-you-sorted-and-filed

Managing the Sweetness Within

My blog covered my experience with infertility before I conceived our son. The specific infertility posts run from early 2006 through August 2006.
www.thesweetnesswithin.blogspot.com

---

*Note: All websites live as of February, 2010.

Notes

The research for this book drew on many sources, both print and online, in person and on paper. Websites and medical studies that support specific statements in each chapter are listed below. I also relied on the following invaluable books for general information about pregnancy, parenthood, infertility, and pregnancy loss: Heidi Murkoff with Sharon Mazel, *What to Expect When You're Expecting*, 4th edition (Workman, 2008); Kathryn Gregorio Palmer, *When You're a Parent With Diabetes: A Real-Life Guide to Staying Healthy While Raising a Family* (HealthyLivingBooks, Hatherleigh, 2006); Diane Aronson and the staff of RESOLVE, *Resolving Infertility* (HarperCollins, 1999); Melissa Ford, *Navigating the Land of IF: Understanding Infertility and Exploring Your Options* (Seal Press, 2009); Julie Vargo and Maureen Regan, *A Few Good Eggs: Two Chicks Dish on Overcoming the Insanity of Infertility* (Regan Books, 2005).

The insight gleaned from online and telephone interviews with medical experts and more than 50 women living with either type 1 or type 2 diabetes provides the foundation for this work, and without them this book would not be what it is.

Chapter 1

1. *Joslin Diabetes Center and Joslin Clinic Guideline for Detection and Management of Diabetes in Pregnancy* (September 14, 2005); Integrated Diabetes Services, *Pregnancy and Type 1 Diabetes Management* (Wynnewood, PA: Integrateddiabetes.com); Lois Jovanovič, "The Importance of Preconception Care in Women with Pre-existing Diabetes," guest editorial, *CADRE's Current Diabetes Practice* 5(2, summer 2006).

2. American Diabetes Association, http://professional.diabetes.org/gluco-secalculator.aspx. See also www.dlife.com/dLife/do/ShowContent/blood_sugar_management/testing/a1c_conversion.html; dLife cites Curt L. Rohlfing et al., "Defining the Relationship Between Plasma Glucose and HbA1c," *Diabetes Care* 25 (2002): 275–8.

3. Dorte M. Jensen et al., "Peri-Conceptional A1C and Risk of Serious Adverse Pregnancy Outcome in 933 Women With Type 1 Diabetes," *Diabetes Care* 32 (2009): 1046–8.

4. O. Langer et al., "Glycemic control in gestational diabetes mellitus—how tight is tight enough: small for gestational age versus large for gestational age?" *American Journal of Obstetrics and Gynecology*, September 1989, 161 (3) 646–653

5. A retrospective study of 73 women (30 with type 1, 43 nondiabetics as controls) at the University of Palermo, Italy, and a study of 115 type 1 women, five type 2 women, and seven women with gestational diabetes in Wycombe, UK, found that glargine did not cause "unexpected adverse maternal or fetal outcome" but recommended further study. See M. P. Imbergamo et al., "Use of Glargine in Pregnant Women With Type 1 Diabetes Mellitus: A Case-Control Study," *Clinical Therapeutics* 30 (2008): 1476–84; I. W. Gallen et al., "Survey of Glargine Use in 115 Pregnant Women With Type 1 Diabetes," *Diabetic Medicine* 25 (2008): 165–9.

6. www.diabetes.org/genetics.jsp.

Chapter 2

1. Deanna Glick, "Diabetes in the Movies: Is Hollywood Shooting in the Dark?" Diabetes Health, November 1, 2002, www.diabeteshealth.com/read/2002/11/01/3036/diabetes-in-the-movies <http://www.diabeteshealth.com/read/2002/11/01/3036/diabetes-in-the-movies>; Steel Magnolias Wikipedia listing, en.wikipedia.org/wiki/Steel_Magnolias <http://en.wikipedia.org/wiki/Steel_Magnolias>

Chapter 3

1. www.marchofdimes.com/pnhec/159_514.asp.
2. www.marchofdimes.com/pnhec/173_15354.asp.
3. www.marchofdimes.com/pnhec/159_9472.asp.
4. www.marchofdimes.com/pnhec/159_514.asp.

5. www.iom.edu/dris. Scroll down and click on the "Macronutrients" table for carbohydrate, protein, and fat intake during pregnancy, and on the "Elements" table for iron intake.
6. www.americanheart.org/presenter.jhtml?identifier=532.
7. www.marchofdimes.com/pnhec/159_823.asp; www.womenshealth. gov/pregnancy/pregnancy/eat.cfm#diet; L. L. Kaiser et al., "Nutrition and Lifestyle for a Healthy Pregnancy Outcome," *Journal of the American Dietetic Association* 102 (2002): 1470–90.
8. www.epa.gov/pesticides/health/human.htm#healtheffects.
9. www.msnbc.msn.com/id/13737389/page/2/a.
10. L. L. Kaiser et al., "Position of the American Dietetic Association: Nutrition and Lifestyle for a Healthy Pregnancy Outcome," *Journal of the American Dietetic Association* 108 (2008): 553–61.
11. www.marchofdimes.com/pnhec/159_826.asp; www.marchofdimes.com/ professionals/14332_1152.asp; www.fda.gov/Food/ResourcesForYou/ HealthEducators/ucm083308.htm.
12. www.glycemicindex.com. Information on low- and high-GI foods is taken from an interview with Emmy Suhl.
13. http://mayoclinic.com/health/morning-sickness/DS01150/ DSECTION=risk%2Dfactors.

Chapter 4

1. www.dol.gov/whd/fmla/fmlaAmended.htm.
2. Information from interviews with Mary Beth Bahren; "Screening for Chromosome Abnormalities" [pamphlet], Beth Israel Deaconess Medical Center, Department of Obstetrics & Gynecology.
3. http://fpb.cwru.edu/Bedrest, the "Pregnancy Bed Rest" website, compiled by Judy Maloni of the Case Western Reserve University School of Nursing. Information was also supplied in phone and email communications with Maloni in November 2009.
4. www.joslin.org/info/diabetic_retinopathy.html.

Chapter 5

1. The information on the super bolus was clarified in email communications with John Walsh. The concept was first referred to as the "super bolus" at the Children With Diabetes conference in

September 2004. It was published as slides 43 through 47 in a slide presentation called "Changes in Diabetes Care, a History of Insulin & Pumps—Past, Present, and Future" by John Walsh; see www.childrenwithdiabetes.com/presentations/DMCare-Past-Future-0904_files/v3_document.htm or www.diabetesnet.com/diabetes_presentations/super-bolus.html. The super bolus is discussed in John Walsh and Ruth Robert, *Pumping Insulin: Everything You Need for Success on a Smart Insulin Pump*, 4th edition (Torrey Pines, 2006), p. 56. It was also evaluated in J. Bondia et al., "Coordinated Basal-Bolus for Tighter Postprandial Glucose Control in Insulin Pump Therapy," *Journal of Diabetes Science and Technology* 2008 (3): 89–97. This mathematical modeling study found that shifting three hours of basal insulin into a bolus could lead to a significant lowering of postprandial glucose levels.

2. Much of the insight in the exercise section comes from Dr. Sheri Colberg, author of the *Diabetic Athlete's Handbook* (Human Kinetics, 2009). See her website, shericolberg.com, for books and more detail about diabetes and exercise. Quotes cited as "writes Dr. Colberg" are reprinted from the *Diabetic Athlete's Handbook*, by Sheri R. Colberg, PhD with permission from Human Kinetics. Quotes cited as "said Dr. Colberg" come from an email interview in August 2009.

Chapter 6

1. L. Molsted-Pedersen and C. Kuhl, "Obstetrical Management in Diabetic Pregnancy: The Copenhagen Experience," *Diabetologia* 1986 (29): 13–16.

2. Grable cited the American College of Obstetricians and Gynecologists' *ACOG Practice Bulletin: Clinical Management Guide lines for Obstetricians-Gynecologists regarding Pregestational Diabetes Mellitus* (Number 60, March 2005). See S. L. Kjos et al., "Insulin-Requiring Diabetes in Pregnancy: A Randomized Trial of Active Induction of Labor and Expectant Management," *American Journal of Obstetrics & Gynecology* 1993 (169): 611–15.

3. Pacifier use may be linked to shorter breastfeeding times. See H. Kronborg and M. Vaeth, "How Are Effective Breastfeeding Technique and Pacifier Use Related to Breastfeeding Problems and Breastfeeding Duration?" *Birth* 2009 (36): 34–42.

4. www.americanpregnancy.org/labornbirth/breechpresentation.html.
5. www.dona.org. On hiring a doula, see www.dona.org/mothers/how_to_hire_a_doula.php.
6. http://birthwhisperer.blogspot.com/2009/10/bullying-of-pregnant-mothers.html.
7. MJ Haller et al. Autologous umbilical cord blood infusion for type 1 diabetes, *Exp Hematol.* 2008 Jun; 36(6): 710–715.

Chapter 7

1. www.dlife.com/dLife/do/ShowContent/inspiration_expert_advice/expert_columns/garnero_0106.html.
2. www.babycenter.com/0_the-apgar-score_3074.bc?page=1.
3. www.mayoclinic.com/health/mrsa/DS00735.

Chapter 8

1. T. C. Takoudes et al., "Risk of Cesarean Wound Complications in Diabetic Gestations," *American Journal of Obstetrics & Gynecology* 2004 (191): 958–63.
2. www.womenshealth.gov/breastfeeding/benefits.
3. http://trigr.epi.usf.edu.
4. http://familydoctor.org/online/famdocen/home/women/pregnancy/ppd/general/379.html; www.mayoclinic.com/health/postpartum-depression/DS00546/DSECTION=symptoms.
5. K. B. Kozhimannil et al., "Association Between Diabetes and Perinatal Depression Among Low-Income Mothers," *Journal of the American Medical Association* 2009 (301): 842–7; www.aafp.org/afp/990415ap/990415e.html
6. http://clinicaltrials.gov/ct2/info/understand#Q02.
7. Karin A. Bilich, "Birth Control While Breastfeeding," *American Baby* magazine, www.parents.com/parenting/relationships/post-partum-birth-control/birth-control-while-breastfeeding/?page=2; American College of Obstetricians and Gynecologists patient education pamphlet on Birth Control, www.acog.org/publications/patient_education/ab020.cfm.
8. www.implanon.com.
9. www.depoprovera.com.
10. www.nuvaring.com/Consumer/index.asp.

11. www.mirena-us.com.
12. http://paragard.com/home.php.

Appendix

1. www.resolve.org/site/PageServer?pagename=lrn_wii_hdik.
2. http://mayoclinic.com/health/female-infertility/DS01053.
3. www.resolve.org/site/PageServer?pagename=lrn_oyf_rfw.
4. M. A. M. Hassan and S. R. Killick, "Effect of Male Age on Fertility: Evidence for the Decline in Male Fertility With Increasing Age," *Fertility and Sterility* 2003 (79): 1520–7.
5. Aronson and the staff of RESOLVE, *Resolving Infertility*; Vargo and Regan, *A Few Good Eggs*; Ford, *Navigating the Land of IF*; www.marchofdimes.com/professionals/14332_1192.asp.

Index